'though born in Easington, County Durham, Les
͗le spent his first eight years in Ratho, south-west
͗inburgh. His father's subsequent career moves led
and his family on a whistle-stop tour of England
b͗re they eventually settled in Birmingham when Les
was in his mid-teens.

He joined Birmingham's Metropolitan Ambulance
͗vice in 1977, for little more reason than it seemed a
͗ood idea at the time. That good idea led to three
͗nbroken decades of round-the-clock emergency work.

Les Pringle is the holder of the Queen's Medal for
Long and Exemplary Service.

Also by Les Pringle

Call the Ambulance!

and published by Corgi Books

Dial 999!

Les Pringle

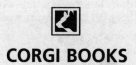

CORGI BOOKS

TRANSWORLD PUBLISHERS
61–63 Uxbridge Road, London W5 5SA
A Random House Group Company
www.transworldbooks.co.uk

DIAL 999!
A CORGI BOOK: 9780552165310

First published in Great Britain
in 2009 by Bantam Press as *Blue Lights and Long Nights*
an imprint of Transworld Publishers
Corgi edition published 2009
Corgi edition reissued as *Dial 999!* 2011

Addresses for Random House Group Ltd companies outside the UK
can be found at: www.randomhouse.co.uk
The Random House Group Ltd Reg. No. 954009

The Random House Group Limited supports The Forest Stewardship Council®
(FSC®), the leading international forest certification organisation. All our titles
that are printed on Greenpeace approved FSC® certified paper carry the FSC®
logo. Our paper procurement policy can be found at
www.randomhouse.co.uk/environment

Typeset in 12/15.5pt Times New Roman by Falcon Oast Graphic Art Ltd.
Printed in the UK by CPI Cox & Wyman, Reading, RG1 8EX.

2 4 6 8 10 9 7 5 3 1

*For Marie-Madeleine, John, Claire
and little Esmée*

With special thanks to Gerard Lynch for his help
and encouragement.

'I've been drinking vodka all my life, sir, and I've never seen a reindeer before. Honestly I haven't.'

Chapter One

In the grey light of early morning it was difficult to make sense of what I was looking at. A man, clad in a dressing gown, appeared to be kneeling on the end of the bed. His body leaned forward slightly with both arms hanging in space. It was a position that defied gravity, making the figure look as if it had been frozen in the act of falling. The chalky whiteness of his skin glowed dully from the shadows but equally unsettling was the utter stillness of the scene. I moved closer and tentatively reached out to take his wrist: it was as cold as a block of marble. I tried to move the fingers, but they were stiff and unyielding. Reluctantly, I looked properly into his face. The eyes and mouth were half open and the lips, white on the edges, had turned a deep purple.

A taut line of cord emerged from somewhere behind his neck, stretching upwards to a hook embedded in a door near the foot of the bed. His knees were resting on the bed but it was the noose that had taken most of his weight. The cord had bitten deep, disappearing into the folds of flesh under his chin and forcing his head slightly to one side. I glanced at Paul, but he just shrugged; there was nothing to be said.

The dead man's landlady had let us into the bedsit a few minutes earlier. She'd been nervous and after pushing open the door had retreated back into the hallway, refusing to go any further. I cast an eye over the little room. What light there was filtered through a solitary window, under which stood a small wooden dining table with a single chair drawn up beneath it. A half-used bottle of tomato sauce sat on a garish tablecloth. On our left was a sideboard with nothing on it save an unused ashtray and a clock. Next to the sideboard was a sink and next to that a two-ring cooker. There were no pictures, not even a mirror hanging against the tired wallpaper; no ornaments, no newspapers or books lying around, no television or radio, not so much as a dirty cup in the sink. The sauce bottle was the only indication that the place might be inhabited. It was more a prison cell ready for inspection than a home.

The dead man's resemblance to Paddy struck me from the start. He was about the same build and height, and had similarly angular features. In fact, the similarity was so uncanny that I made a mental note to tell Paddy when I saw him in the pub later that night. It would be the blackest of humour, but I could picture his wry smile if I were to go one step further and suggest that, for a moment, I had thought it was him hanging there. Then the sound of Paul rummaging through a drawer in the bedside table distracted me and I turned to see what he'd found. He was flicking through the pages of a building society passbook, looking for a clue to the man's identity.

'This has to be him, I suppose.' He read out a name. It didn't mean anything to me, but I wasn't paying attention. Something was wrong. Something was gnawing at the back of my mind, leaving me feeling slightly sick. I moved closer to the body and looked carefully into the face for a second time. Paddy? No, surely not. It was too silly. I stepped back and checked from a different angle and, as I did so, my stomach turned to water.

'Oh God. Paddy . . . what have you done?'

This couldn't be happening. Paddy, the Aston Villa fan, would be in the pub tonight as usual. This was a dream. In desperation I looked to Paul, as if hoping he would tell me that it was all a big mistake. He stared back.

'What's wrong? Did you know him?'

His use of the past tense broke the spell and I sank heavily on to the wooden chair by the table. I tried to focus on the tomato sauce bottle.

'Yes, I know him.'

The darkest thought lurking in the mind of anyone working for the ambulance service is that one day you may be called to a friend or relative. Paddy wasn't a close friend, but close enough.

The pub was the only place we ever met. He would always be in the same spot, propping up the bar with a pint of Guinness at his elbow. From this vantage point he could survey the room and nod and smile at people as they came and went. He never seemed tempted to sit down with the regulars for a chat. Not that anyone took offence; it was accepted without comment that that was the way he was. It was enough for him to hear a chorus of 'Hello, Paddy' when he arrived, and 'Good night, Paddy' when he left. When someone did engage him in a snatched conversation at the bar, he would straighten up his tall, gaunt frame, smile and be perfectly affable. Yet, despite his easy-going disposition, there was no mistaking the loner in him. He was at one with the bustle and camaraderie the pub provided, albeit on his own terms.

In the three or four years I'd known him, I'd grown to like him, and had come to enjoy our brief conversations about football or whatever else took our fancy. But now guilt crept through my shock as I thought back to when I had last seen him, only a couple of days earlier. Had there been a clue? Something I'd missed? There must have been. Then again, if I had noticed something, what could I have done or said that might have stopped him doing this? There were no answers. I would never know why he found death preferable to life but perhaps the small, empty world of his bedsit spoke for him. The pub was his real home. It was probably the only place in the world that offered him a sense of belonging, with the public bar the closest thing to a living room he'd known in adult life. But even there he was effectively anonymous. To my shame, I hadn't even known his real name.

I was calmer now but couldn't shake off the despondency that had enveloped me. What was I doing here? Why had I chosen a career that would inevitably lead me to confront events that most rational people would do anything to avoid? Years of asking myself the same question has delivered precious few answers, and none of them satisfactory. If I look back to my life before joining the ambulance service there are no clues to what motivated me, only a chain of thoughts that can be traced to a freezing afternoon in Edinburgh a lifetime ago.

Chapter Two

Had it been an old Hollywood movie, the bartender would have put down the bourbon glass he was polishing, flicked the towel over his shoulder and sidled up to lend me a sympathetic ear. But it wasn't Hollywood, it was Edinburgh, so the barman remained on his stool reading the rugby page with a roll-up glued to his lower lip. If I'd had a shoulder to cry on things might have turned out differently but, as it was, the further down my pint I got, the further I sank into melancholy. My surroundings didn't help much. Maybe I wasn't very good at choosing pubs, but this place had all the ambience of a British Rail waiting room.

I ordered another pint and looked for something to grumble about. Football! Oh how I missed English football. Watching the likes of Partick Thistle play Ayr United on TV lost its appeal when you knew Manchester United v Arsenal was being shown down south. Then there was the rest of Scottish television.

Back in the seventies, a biopic on Andy Stewart or *An Evening with Jimmy Shand and His Band* was about as good as it got. Documentaries chronicling ruddy-cheeked crofters plucking gannets' eggs from cliff-face nests might be some people's cup of tea, but they weren't mine. What with the weather, no wonder the entire nation was planning to emigrate, or was in the pub, or was screaming from Presbyterian pulpits.

I took a sip of beer and hunched down into my pub coat in the hope of finding a bit of warmth. Pub coats were essential if you were thinking of spending more than five minutes in an Edinburgh bar during the winter of '76. With their cold lino floors, luke-warm radiators and chilled, fizzy beer, you needed the constitution of Scott of the Antarctic to feel at home in one. Mind you, it was even worse outside. A couple of hours earlier I'd set off to visit a customer in the nearby town of Duns, only to be driven back to the city by a blizzard the like of which I wouldn't have dreamed possible outside Alaska. Faced with the choice of catching up on some paperwork back at the office or nipping into the pub for a quick one, I chose the pub. As things turned out, it proved to be a pretty significant decision.

When I took delivery of a third pint the unexpected happened . . . I began to mellow. I felt a little warmer, and even undid the top two buttons of my coat. I wasn't being fair on Edinburgh, or Scotland for that matter. When Marie and I arrived as newlyweds in the late summer it had been beautiful. It wasn't anybody's fault this was one of the worst winters in living memory. What I needed more than anything to lift my spirits was some warmth, some sunshine even.

By the time the fourth pint was pushed in front of me I was fantasizing about abandoning everything and running off to the south of France. It wasn't a new day-dream; it had been finding its way into my mind more and more in recent days. This time, though, it took on a new twist.

Why don't you just do it, I thought. Go to France. What's to stop you?

Well, loads of things. There was my career for a start: it was the reason Marie and I had moved up to Scotland in the first place. I was twenty-three, newly married and after two years' training was holding down a well-paid job in the paper trade. The idea of giving it up and running off to the Riviera was nothing short of madness. I would be throwing away all I'd worked for.

The inner voice, or maybe it was the inner beer, hadn't finished with me:

Nonsense! Do you really want a career that, if it doesn't bore you to death first, will at best culminate in a respectable semi at the end of a cul-de-sac forty years from now? Of course you don't. You've got to find something completely different, something better. Something that'll give you a bit of satisfaction.

But what?

Then it came to me. A few days earlier I'd been listening to *Woman's Hour* on the car radio. The

18

programme had been running a series of ten-minute talks in which people described their jobs and why they loved them so much. On this particular day it was the turn of a London ambulance man. He was a jolly-voiced chap and the picture he painted sounded rather alluring: job satisfaction, responsibility, decision-making, variety, not sitting in an office and, best of all, no bosses breathing down your neck. Being an ambulance man had an air of respectability about it; not high status perhaps, but a solid, honest feel. I put down my pint and smiled at the idea of racing around in an ambulance. It was too ridiculous. But the more I turned it over in my head, the less outrageous it seemed.

This was a pleasant way to kill time in the pub and I returned to the thought of lazing around on a Mediterranean beach. I'm not sure if the expression 'gap year' existed in those days, but even if it did I wasn't eligible as I hadn't been to university. No, if this fantasy were to be lived out it would have to be conducted as a kind of post-hippie gesture. A trip with no agenda, a trip where we could go and do whatever we wanted. Marie and I could give notice to our employers; sell all our possessions . . . Hang on, other than clothes we didn't have any possessions worth talking about. Things like my pub coat, scarves, gloves, woollen hats, hot-water bottles, blankets and my cantankerous paraffin heater, we could give to a charity shop. In Edinburgh, they'd fly out the door in minutes. The car belonged to the company and the flat was rented, so they weren't a problem. I didn't know how much we had in the bank, but I thought it must be a reasonable amount. If we took a tent and got around by hitchhiking we could last ages.

By way of nudging the dream one step further, I began to wonder what Marie would say if I brought up the subject. I started by assuming she would give it short shrift, but then thought otherwise.

For one thing, she felt the cold more than me. When the plunging temperatures turned my nose red back in November, hers had turned blue. Her 1960s Afghan coat might have been OK for the Khyber Pass, but it was no match for an Edinburgh winter. Then there was her job. She worked for a scatterbrained character whose business talents seemed confined to dodging phone calls and staying one step ahead of the bailiffs. I never did understand exactly what kind of set-up he was trying to run, but I knew Marie spent most of her time either fending off dissatisfied customers or placating irate creditors. The loss of this job wouldn't cause her any heartache. And there was something else; something that could only be regarded as my trump card . . . She was French. Surely she would jump at the chance to show me round her country?

I undid the last couple of buttons on my coat and ordered what I admit was a completely unnecessary final pint. While I watched the barman trying to control a geyser of froth spilling over the glass my thoughts returned to the ambulance service. Was it such a mad idea? The answer came back with such startling clarity that it shocked me. No, it wasn't a mad idea, it was nothing short of inspirational and, what's more, it was exactly what I was going to do. The realization that a daydream had somehow become a conviction made me slightly weak at the knees. Was I really going to give up my job, clear off to France and join the ambulance service when I got back? You bet I was, and nothing would stop me.

I looked round the bar as if fearing someone might have noticed the change in me. I needn't have worried. The barman, having managed to fill my glass, was now engrossed in page three and the only other occupants of the room, an old man and his dog, appeared to be asleep. Gazing through the window, I watched the north-easterly wind chase a blanket of orange-grey clouds across the sky and felt a warm glow spread through me. Yes, I thought. Watch out, St Tropez; move over, Brigitte Bardot, I'm on my way.

It didn't take long to chip the ice from Marie's initial reaction to my plan. After all, how often would such a chance come along? We had no dependants, no debts or commitments, we didn't even have a pot plant to worry about; we were beholden to nobody but ourselves. And, still in that happy frame of mind, we heaved on our rucksacks and headed south a few weeks later. France was all I hoped it would be and St Tropez didn't disappoint either, but I'm sorry to say Brigitte Bardot did.

Maybe she was in Edinburgh for the festival; wherever she was, she didn't turn up on our beach. Not that I let it spoil things. For the next few months we lazed around with the other beach bums in a life of blissful idleness.

It couldn't last for ever, of course, and as the summer drifted into late September the campsite began to thin out. At first we tried to ignore the patches of dead grass left by the missing tents but soon there was no getting away from it: the people we had come to know as friends were upping sticks and heading home. Arriving back in England with only a suntan and a tent riddled with cigarette holes would present its own problems, but what the heck. Two safety nets were in place. One was the spare room in my parents' house in Birmingham, and the other was the reasonable wedge of cash still lodged with the Royal Bank of Scotland. We had managed to hold on to this money by being extraordinarily frugal over the last few months, to the point where sharing an omelette in a café felt decadent. More importantly, time hadn't weakened my resolve to join the ambulance service. I'd given it plenty of thought and was keener than ever to have a crack at it.

The return journey through France was marked by a prophetic event. We had hitched a lift and were travelling along a particularly winding and narrow road when the car was brought to a halt by a queue of stationary vehicles. Coming across a traffic jam on a little-used B-road was odd and, after sitting there for a few minutes, I decided to stretch my legs and find out what was holding us up. I had only covered about twenty yards when the road swung right and dis-appeared behind a hedgerow. Ahead of me, people were out of their cars and gathered on the bend to watch whatever was going on. When I reached them I saw the problem. The rear end of a small red hatchback was sticking out of the drainage ditch running along-side the road, with what looked like a breakdown truck parked close by. It was only when I read *Sapeur Pompiers – Véhicule de secours* written along its length that I realized it was an ambulance and that this was something serious.

There was movement inside the car and the body of a young man was lifted out and laid on a waiting stretcher. Next came the body of a young woman. I was dumbfounded. Stupidly, I looked round at the others as if expecting to be told that it was all part of a training exercise, but no one spoke. The image of those few moments on a back road in rural France etched itself on my brain. I remember the girl in particular. She was about nineteen with long chestnut hair and wearing white trousers with red shoes. Her eyes were open and, as they moved her, her head lolled gently one way then the other. There wasn't a mark on her, nor on her companion. Neither carried any outward evidence of what had killed them.

I wasn't aware of the hollow feeling that had crept into my chest until I retraced my steps down the line of cars and found that I couldn't breathe evenly. My head was spinning. Who were they? Where were they going? Why were they dead? Silly questions, but they kept coming. Were they friends or lovers? Brother and sister? Were they arguing or laughing at the last moment? Most of all, how could two young lives be snuffed out in the blink of an eye? Over the next few days I fell into gloomy introspection and kept re-examining my response to what I'd seen. An hour wouldn't pass without my mind drifting back. Red shoes. Why did I keep seeing her red shoes? It threw my plans for joining the ambulance service into stark relief. It also forced me to re-examine my motives, which now seemed rather shallow.

The next day I did something I'd never done before, and haven't done since. I went to Poitiers cathedral and lit two candles for two people I never knew.

Chapter Three

It would be foolish to pretend that the accident in France didn't test my resolve. I'd hated what I'd seen, and viewed it as a brutal portent of where my chosen path might lead. And yet, when the mist cleared, I was able to appreciate that joining the ambulance service would offer far more positive aspects than negative. I don't mean that some vague, altruistic calling was behind my decision to soldier on; it just felt right. And with the goal firmly set I wasn't going to be deflected by anything. Given my determination, I was surprised to find my self-confidence ebbing away in the chill morning air as I waited outside my local ambulance station in Sutton Coldfield, just outside Birmingham. What if there were no vacancies? I hadn't even thought of that until now. And, even if there were vacancies, who was to say I'd be offered one? The possibility of rejection hadn't crossed my mind either.

Grappling with these worries made me ridiculously

nervous. It wasn't as if I was there for an interview, I'd only called round to ask for a job application form. None the less, by the time the door opened and a stocky little man in uniform stuck his head out I was ready to bolt.

'Hello . . . can I help you?'

I mumbled something about an application form and watched his face crease into a smile.

'Come in, son. I should be able to sort you one out.'

I stepped inside and waited while he dropped the latch. He was well into middle age with heavily Brylcreemed hair, a weatherbeaten face and, if the way he moved was anything to go by, an arthritic hip. Not someone to feature on a recruitment poster perhaps but, in terms of enthusiasm, he proved priceless.

'I'm Bill, by the way,' he said.

'Les Pringle,' I said. 'Nice to meet you.'

He looked me up and down as we shook hands. 'I suppose you'll want to have a look round the place while you're here.'

'Oh, no, I don't want to be a bother.'

'It's no bother, son. We'll just pop into the messroom and get the tea organized first.'

The messroom was a pretty simple affair: a large table in the centre with a few upright chairs, an algae-coated fish tank, a television and, in the far corner, four armchairs, two of which were occupied by men in uniform. Both had their feet up and their eyes closed. Bill viewed them with disdain.

'Bloody hell! What's this, the dead centre of town? There's more life in that bloody fish tank than there is in you two!'

One of the men opened an eye as Bill waved an arm in my direction.

'We've got a visitor. This is . . . er . . .'

'Les,' I offered.

'This is Les. He's thinking of joining and wants to have a look round. I told him you'd put the kettle on, Tony.'

I was startled. 'No, really, I don't want to be a nuisance.'

The man in the chair had both eyes open now. 'You haven't signed anything, have you, mate?'

'Well, no. I've just got here.'

'That's good, because you're making a big mistake. Take my advice and get out now while you still have the chance.'

Bill looked at me with a resigned expression. 'Ignore him, mucker. It's just that Tony thinks he's got a sense of humour.'

Bill was a Leading Ambulanceman, or LA. This put him on a par with a works foreman, in that he acted as a bridge between road staff and management. His enthusiasm for the service was boundless. I followed him on a depot inspection that covered every nook and cranny. Nothing was left out; he even lifted the lid on the dirty linen basket and invited me to take a look inside, as if it contained some culinary delight. When we emerged from the blanket storeroom there was only one thing left to see. So far Bill had studiously avoided going anywhere near it, but now he led me over to the centre of the garage where the ambulance stood gleaming under the electric lights.

'This,' he said proudly, 'is a Bedford J1 weighing in at three and a half tonnes. It's one of the last of its line, and came out of the Luton works in 1975.' Moving round to the front, he reached up and fondly patted the huge bonnet. 'Under here is a 3,600 cc six-cylinder engine. It does about twelve to the gallon and with a fair wind it'll notch up 70 mph.'

I stood back and took in the sleek lines. In its ivory livery with a single red strip running down the side it looked solid and dependable, more a place of sanctuary than a vehicle.

'Shall we have a look inside, mucker?' Bill, I discovered later, wasn't too good with names and called everyone mucker. He dropped the back step. 'A Hanlan interior. Bedford make the actual vehicle, but Hanlan does the fitting out for us.'

My immediate impression was of cosy security. The floor was a deep red lino flecked with grey, and the walls were a soft cream. A stretcher, made up with a white sheet and red blankets, sat on the left of the aisle, and on the opposite side another stretcher was used as a bench seat with drop-down armrests and padding on the wall behind. Cupboards were squeezed in everywhere they could be squeezed. Bill worked his way along them, pulling out pieces of equipment and explaining their function as he went. Now and then he would purse his lips in disapproval at something that was out of place, but he didn't let it disturb the flow.

'Now!' He held up what looked like a black plastic corset. 'This is a brilliant piece of kit. It's called the Heinz collar.' He looked at it wistfully. 'I suppose with a name like that it must be German. Anyway, not to worry, it's a cervical collar with built-in head and back support for neck injuries. Here, do you want to try it on? It'll give you a better idea of how it works.'

In a matter of seconds I was immobilized. A collar supported by a rigid length of plastic stretching from my chin to my breastbone held my neck firmly in place, while at the back another sheet of rigid plastic ran from the top of my head down to the middle of my back. Straps fastening across the front connected the whole thing.

'Can't move your head or shoulders, can you?'

'No,' I admitted through clenched teeth.

'I can tell you a little story about the Heinz if you want to hear it.'

My attempted nod turned into a bow.

'It happened a couple of summers ago when we were called out to a car crash in town.'

I lowered myself gingerly on to the edge of the bench seat as he continued.

'It was more of a shunt than a crash really. The couple in the car were over here on holiday from

Canada. He was a retired doctor and wasn't hurt, but his wife had a bit of sensitivity in her neck. So I got out the Heinz and was about to slip it into position when he asked me what I thought I was doing. Funny kind of question coming from a doctor, you might think, and even when I tried to explain he didn't want to listen. He said he'd already checked her and reckoned it was only mild whiplash. Well, this put me on the spot. He was a doctor and was probably right, but on the other hand you can't be too careful with necks, can you?'

'No, of course not,' I agreed, trying to appear knowledgeable.

'Anyway,' Bill continued, 'the only person that really mattered was the woman herself so I put it to her that, just to be on the safe side, she should let me fit the Heinz and then come with us to have her neck X-rayed. Her husband wasn't too pleased. Don't get me wrong, he wasn't rude or anything, but he made it clear that he thought our treatment was way over the top.'

Bill smiled at me and seemed to be waiting for a prompt.

'So how was she in the end?' I asked.

'We dropped her off at Casualty and didn't hear anything after that.'

I scratched an itch under the rigid collar while I tried to figure out what the point of this little story was.

'I suppose you're wondering what the point is,' Bill said. 'The point is that two or three months later we got a letter from the woman's husband in Canada. I tell you what, when I read it you could have knocked me over with a feather. He started off by apologizing for being a pain in the arse at the time of the accident, and then spent the rest of the letter praising us for the way we looked after his wife.'

'Why would he do that?'

'Because,' Bill paused dramatically, 'because his wife had only broken her neck in two places.'

'Wow,' I said. 'That must have made you feel good. I don't mean it was good that her neck was broken,' I added hurriedly, 'I mean good that you stuck to your guns and used the Heinz.'

Bill smiled. 'That's why this is such a great job, mucker. Every now and then you get the chance to do something that matters. Anyway, what's left to show you?'

He looked round and spotted a fearsome machine of bellows and hoses sitting on the bulkhead shelf.

'Ah, the Automan,' he said with relish, 'you'll like this. The idea behind this little beauty is to force oxygen into the patient's lungs, leaving you free to do cardiac massage.' Not content with a verbal description, Bill pulled the mask over his face and fixed it in position with the retaining straps. With everything ready, he held up an index finger to ensure my attention and switched on the oxygen. There was a *thunk*, followed by a hissing sigh as the pressurized gas raced out and filled the bellows. When they were fully extended, a metallic *clack* signalled the release of an internal spring and they descended with a whoosh. Bill's cheeks bulged and his eyes widened as he fought the first powerful rush of oxygen. Undaunted, and seemingly unaware that I couldn't make out a word he was saying, he continued his lecture through the rubber facemask. Normally I would have tried to feign understanding by throwing in the occasional well-timed nod, but the Heinz held me like a vice and all I could do was sit bolt upright and watch. I think he was demonstrating cardiac massage when the tea arrived.

I rotated at the hips and thanked Tony as he placed the mugs on the back step. He stared at us impassively for a second or two, and then shook his head.

'Bill, I swear to God,' he said in a voice loud enough to be heard over the hissing and clacking of the Automan, 'they're going to come and take you away one day, and I hope I'm around to watch when they do.'

With the long canvas hose swaying in front of him, Bill leaned over and switched off the oxygen supply.

'You say something?'

'Yeah.' Tony gave me a surreptitious wink. 'Why have you got this poor kid done up like he's about to be delivered to the loony bin while you're sitting there playing bomber pilots?'

Bill pulled off the rubber facemask and looked at me.

'You see what I have to put up with, mucker? There's no respect any more. That's the trouble with the service these days. Now let's get you out of

32

that contraption and find that bloody application form.'

The station office was a small room dominated by a large wooden desk covered with bits of paper and teacups. Bill swung himself confidently into the chair and started rummaging through the drawers. After a couple of fruitless minutes, frustration began to take over.

'You see! This is the kind of problem I have to deal with, mucker. You set up a system so that everyone knows exactly where everything is, and by the time you come back on duty some daft bugger's changed it all round.' He slammed the final drawer shut and put on a pair of glasses before crossing to an ancient filing cabinet. 'People just can't leave things alone. If I had my way . . . Hang on . . . Here we are!' He pulled out a form from a recess that probably hadn't seen the light of day for months.

'This is the chap you want.' He passed it across. 'If you fill it out, I'll make sure it goes in the internal post this afternoon.'

I glanced at the form while Bill cleared a corner of the desk for me. It didn't ask for very much; in fact it asked for very little. Apart from the space set aside for my name, address and date of birth, there was a box for my employment history and another for any qualifications I might have.

'Er, Bill,' I said, 'these boxes aren't very big.'

'Oh?'

'I've got seven O-levels,' I said, 'and there's no way I can fit them into this little box.'

Bill looked over my shoulder. 'Mm, I see what you mean. You'll just have to squeeze in as many as you can. Don't worry about the rest.'

'Can't I attach them on a separate piece of paper?'

'Nah. It'll only get lost. Anyway, three will be more than enough.'

Those O-levels hadn't come easily, but I gave up without a fight and jotted down what I thought were the three most relevant: human biology, sociology and English.

The other four might as well have gone in the bin. Bill took the form, sealed it in an envelope and tossed it into a tray on the desk.

'There you go, mucker, done and dusted. Don't hold your breath waiting for a reply. Our lot aren't the quickest off the blocks when it comes to correspondence.'

Leaning back in the chair, he clasped his hands behind his head and took on a wistful look.

'You know, you calling in like this has got me thinking back. When I was a youngster like you, my station superintendent had to go up the local high street on Saturday mornings with a clipboard and try to recruit people. Can you imagine having to do that now? Mind you, the poor bastard was on a hiding to nothing. The wages were crap compared to the local factories.'

I was tempted to point out that the wages were still crap, but thought better of it.

'Of course,' Bill continued, 'the people who joined

in those days were committed to the job. In fact, it wasn't a job then, it was a way of life. You don't get any sense of vocation from youngsters these days – I doubt if half of them could even spell the word. All they want to do is race round the streets playing with the sirens.' He took his eyes off the ceiling and looked at me. 'There weren't even bells on the ambulances when I started, mucker, never mind sirens. I still remember the man coming to fit the bells like it was yesterday . . .'

An hour or so later I was on the bus home. That visit to the station might have been a small step, but it set a course that was to map out the rest of my life.

Chapter Four

A week later I received a letter inviting me to report for a driving test at Henrietta Street Ambulance Station. If Bill had seduced me into thinking everyone in the service was friendly and welcoming, then Warren Harris clearly saw it as his duty to redress the balance. Podgy, in his mid-forties with thinning hair, he exuded all the charm of a Bolivian border guard.

'Mr Pringle, isn't it?'

'Yes, that's right.'

'Good.' He drew out the word distractedly and shuffled some papers on his desk before glancing at his watch.

'Nice to see you're on time. Driving licence, please.'

I passed it over and waited while he studied it with the meticulous care of someone tipped off to expect a forgery. It was only as he handed it back that he looked me in the eye for the first time.

'I have to warn you that your application to join the

service won't go any further unless I'm satisfied your driving meets the required standard. The test will take about twenty minutes. Before we go out to the vehicle there are two things for you to remember. Firstly, you will follow the road, and only deviate if I instruct you to turn left or right. Is that clear?'

'Yes.'

'Secondly, and this is important,' he leaned forward slightly, 'if at any time you give me cause to lose confidence in your driving ability, or should you mount the pavement, the test will be over and I will drive the vehicle back to station.'

Mount the pavement? Why on earth would I mount the pavement?

'Do you have any questions?'

'No, I don't think so,' I said meekly.

He regarded me from an expressionless face. 'You didn't consider having a haircut then?'

This caught me off guard. I'd thought he might quiz me on my driving experience but not on the length of my hair, especially as I'd made a point of getting it cut the previous day. It couldn't have been more than a couple of inches over my collar, which by the standards of the day was tantamount to a scalping.

'Well actually, I did go—'

'A bit late to worry about it now.' He stood up and reached for his cap. 'If you can manage to see the road through it, I'll have to settle for that.'

I followed him out across the garage to an elderly

ambulance parked away from the others. It was a sad sight. Doubtless the pride of the fleet once upon a time, it now looked tired and careworn . . . as if all it wanted was to be left alone. The paintwork had lost its sheen, the wheel arches were pitted with rust, even the tyres seemed to sag. I was casting a dubious eye over some recent repair work to the front wing when Mr Harris opened the driver's door.

'Come on then, in you get. I've got a meeting at eleven.'

Climbing two steps up into the cab, I gazed over the huge steering wheel at the world below with mounting trepidation. I'd never been in a vehicle this big, let alone driven one. My examiner sat beside me on the bench seat.

'If the wing mirrors are set properly, start her up.'

I waggled the three-foot-long gearstick to make sure we were in neutral and turned the ignition key. The engine coughed and burped but, after three or four seconds of trying, didn't show any inclination to start. I switched off, and was about to have another go when Mr Harris snapped, 'Choke! Give her some choke, lad! You've got a choke on your own car, haven't you? The lever's down on your right.'

With the choke lever fully out, all six cylinders caught and the cab began to rattle and throb to the beat of the engine. Mr Harris raised his voice.

'Now, drive to the main doors. If it's clear, turn left . . .'

He didn't get any further. A shriek of tortured metal erupted from under the bonnet as I pushed the gearstick forward.

'No! No!' He was near panic-stricken. 'Are you trying to wreck the gearbox? There's no synchromesh on first gear! You've got to let the revs fall off before engaging it! If you're looking for mod cons on this old girl I've got news for you: you won't bloody well find any.'

My neck went hot. He was shouting at me already, and we hadn't even moved.

I took my foot off the accelerator and tried to regain some composure before pushing down the heavy clutch again. It slipped smoothly into gear this time but that didn't prevent a world-weary sigh coming from my left.

'You're going to flood her.'

'Pardon me?'

'You're going to flood the carburettor if you don't let the choke in.' He took off his glasses and rubbed his eyes. 'I really shouldn't have to tell you these things, you know.'

'Sorry.' I fumbled for the lever. Determined to stay cool, I maintained gentle pressure on the accelerator and carefully eased out the clutch until I felt it bite. Confident that things were now coming back under my control, I reached for the handbrake and pulled. Nothing happened; it wouldn't budge. I heaved with all my strength but the wretched thing might as well have been welded in position. My new-found cool evaporated and in the struggle my foot slipped off the clutch. We lurched forward a couple of feet as the engine stalled with a clang that echoed round the garage.

The ensuing silence hung heavy in the cab. After a few moments, and not daring to look at Mr Harris, I mumbled, 'Sorry, but I seem to have a problem with the handbrake.' When there was no immediate response I darted a glance in his direction. He was sitting with pursed lips, looking contemplative.

'I think I know what's happened here,' he said, more to himself than to me. 'And if I'm right someone's going to swing for it!' He leaned over and gave the handbrake a fierce tug. When that didn't work he brought both arms to bear and pulled until he was red in the face. After a few seconds he gave up and sat back in the seat with a sigh.

'It's got to be one of those bloody clowns on "C" shift. It's absolutely typical of their juvenile mentality.'

I couldn't be sure what he was getting at, but I saw a glimmer of hope.

'You don't mean someone's deliberately pulled the brake on so tight as some kind of joke, do you?' I tried to sound indignant.

'That's exactly what I mean. Stupid pranks are something you'll have to get used to if you end up working here. It must have got out that I was taking someone for a test this morning ... and this is the result. Infantile, that's what it is. Infantile.'

After releasing the handbrake by crouching on the seat and pulling with both hands, I started her up again. A dense plume of black smoke belched from the exhaust and we chugged slowly across the garage and out on to the road. I didn't know what to expect of the 'old girl', but it didn't take long to find out she had the handling qualities of a combine harvester. Any illusions I'd harboured that this might be my chance to show off some innate driving skills were forgotten as the next twenty minutes degenerated into a trial of strength.

Throughout my ordeal Mr Harris sat with his hands clasped on his lap, silently staring through the windscreen. Apart from the occasional 'Turn left' or 'Turn right', he didn't say a word. I had a sneaking feeling that he was more interested in plotting his revenge on 'C' shift than in keeping too close an eye on me. For my part, I concentrated on not mounting the pavement. My reward for making it back to station without notching up a single pedestrian was to be told that my driving, while leaving plenty of scope for improvement, met the basic requirements laid down by the service.

The way was now clear for a formal interview the following week. It proved to be a fairly perfunctory affair lasting no more than fifteen minutes, five of which were taken up by a lively debate on the length of my hair. When it was over we all shook hands and I was told that, subject to another haircut, I would receive a formal letter offering me a position. Things were going better than I could have hoped. Two days earlier Marie had been offered a secretarial job with a medical agency and now, within a month of being back in the country, the final part of the plan had fallen into place.

My contract of employment arrived by post a week later. I would have to complete a twelve-month probationary period during which I would receive the necessary training and front-line experience. A six-week residential course was starting the following Monday. I was to report to the central fire brigade headquarters, where a couple of rooms in the attic had been put at our disposal. That's not exactly how they worded it but that was what it amounted to. The service apparently didn't have any facilities of its own and was forced to rent training space. So there it was: my first six weeks with the ambulance service would be spent in a fire brigade attic.

Most of the dozen or so people on the course were in their mid- to late twenties and, like me, had no real idea of what they were letting themselves in for. None of us had even the most tenuous experience in health care. Among others, there was a technician from the GPO, a bookie, a council gardener, the manager of a newsagent's shop, a mechanic and a sadly disillusioned maths teacher. On the face of it we didn't have a great deal in common other than a willingness to abandon our previous jobs and jump head first into the unknown. And it really was the unknown. Back in the seventies there wasn't the present-day plethora of fly-on-the-wall documentaries and medical dramas on television to inspire people. I remember watching *Emergency-Ward 10* as a child, but all that did was give me a morbid fear of one day being incarcerated in an iron lung while a nurse and junior doctor conducted an illicit affair just out of my vision. Any notion of what it might be like to work on an ambulance came entirely from the imagination.

Both instructors assigned to our course were likeable and enthusiastic, but that was about as far as any similarity went. Mike Phillips was the kind of bloke you would quite happily spend an evening with in the pub. Personable, with an easy laugh, he never took himself or anything else too seriously. Gerald Hastings, on the other hand, took everything very seriously. I'd never met anyone so completely devoid of a sense of humour as Gerald. He was pleasant and attentive, but when confronted by light-hearted banter or, heaven forbid, a joke, he was left floundering, and he would look up in alarm when something amused the group and a trickle of laughter crossed the room.

Mike concentrated on the practical side of our training, which left Gerald the task of trying to bang home the theory. This was fine by me. Of the O-levels I managed to pass, human biology was by far the toughest. At the time it seemed a lot of effort for very little purpose, but now I found myself reaping the unforeseen benefits. While Gerald droned on about the various body systems, I was able to sit back and watch out for the occasional cloud to drift past the attic window.

On the practical side, we bandaged and splinted each other interminably in all kinds of imaginary scenarios. Pressure points caused me particular concern. These are precise areas of the body where external pressure can be applied over an artery to stop the blood flow. Useful knowledge if you come across someone bleeding to death. The problem was that we couldn't practise on each other. People don't like having their arteries squashed, so it had to remain a theoretical exercise in the hope that it would all come together in a real-life emergency. I was particularly spooked by a little talk Gerald gave on the subject. As usual, he got off to an enigmatic start.

'A sensible butcher will always wear a chain-mail apron when cutting meat. True?' A glance at our vacant faces prompted him to continue. 'Well, let me tell you . . . it's only a foolish butcher who doesn't wear a chain-mail apron. As we know, broken glass and knives are the arteries' worst enemies, and the preponderance of knives in a butcher's shop leaves him particularly liable to an unfortunate accident. Take the paring knife, for example. Its long, thin blade is razor-sharp, and is usually used in a downward cutting action.' He broke off to simulate this by taking a vicious swipe at the desk. 'If the aim isn't true, there's every chance that the blade will glance off the table and stab the unfortunate butcher somewhere on the inner thigh.' He punched at his own thigh just in case we didn't get the picture. 'And which artery runs through the pelvis and branches into each leg?' Nobody had a chance to answer. 'Yes, that's right, the femoral artery. So, given that the worst has happened, the artery has been punctured and blood is pumping three feet into the air, what do you do when you arrive?'

Roger filled the ensuing silence. 'Get a mop and bucket?'

I'd taken a liking to Roger early on in the course. There was a healthy irreverence about him that I found refreshing; the problem was he didn't quite know where to draw the line. Gerald looked at him in mystification, and then his eyebrows came together in understanding.

'I don't think making light of a serious subject is an appropriate response, Mr Timmins. You might not want to learn anything but I'm sure the others do.' He turned to the rest of us. 'Has anyone got something sensible to say?'

'I would try and stop the bleeding,' came from the back of the room.

'Yes, of course. Stopping the bleeding is the obvious priority. How would that be achieved?'

'I would apply pressure to the femoral artery,' said the same voice.

'Yes, our good old friend the femoral artery. The problem we have is that the only place we can get at it is high up near the groin.' He pointed at a diagram on the board. 'You will have to estimate its position and apply intense pressure to force it against the femur and cut off the bleeding. And don't forget, the pressure has to be maintained until you reach the hospital – no easy task.'

'How long has the butcher got from when he stabs himself?' someone asked.

'Good question,' said Gerald. 'It's hard to be precise, but maybe less than five or six minutes.'

'So he's pretty well had it by the time we get there,' Roger said.

Gerald thought about it. 'Well, his condition will certainly be degrading by the moment, no doubt about that. And there's something else you should be aware of. As you all know, blood transports oxygen to the brain, so when the blood volume is reduced, so are the oxygen levels. In extreme cases this brings on a condition known as hypoxia, which can cause the patient to behave irrationally before he passes out.'

'What do you mean by that?' asked another voice.

'Without enough oxygen to the brain, the patient loses the power to think clearly. He becomes disorientated and might even become aggressive, or abusive.' Gerald was in full flow now. 'The general lack of oxygen also brings on what we call "air hunger". This will instil in the patient an overwhelming sensation that he's being suffocated. The terror of this feeling, coupled with the hypoxia, may cause him to see you as an aggressor and he might try to fight you off with what strength he has left.' He looked solemnly round the group. 'Makes you wonder if you've picked the right job, doesn't it?'

A long silence followed, broken again by Roger. 'At least his mates will have got some good black pudding out of it.'

Gerald eyed him cautiously. 'Black pudding?'

'Yes,' Roger said. 'You know, all that blood . . . great for black pudding if you're a butcher.'

Gerald, to his credit, only twitched.

That night I woke from a dream in which I had been grappling with an eighteen-stone blood-soaked butcher. He'd taken exception to me groping at his groin and wouldn't listen when I tried to tell him it was for his own good.

One skill I failed to acquire was the art of tying effective knots. To this day I don't know why it was part of the syllabus anyway; it wasn't as if we were ever likely to find ourselves rescuing people from mineshafts or mountainsides. No matter how hard I concentrated, and despite Mike Phillips showing patience beyond the call of duty, I failed to see the light. In desperation he would stand in front of me with a length of rope and slowly create a slipknot you would trust on the north face of the Eiger. When I tried, the resulting tangle usually had to be cut from the rope with a pair of scissors. I accidentally got it right on about the hundredth attempt, and Mike gleefully ticked me off as being competent in knots. He was good like that.

Gerald, on the other hand, tended to be less forgiving. Before starting a lecture his habit was to steeple his hands under his chin, fix his gaze somewhere on the ceiling, and pose an introductory question to the group. So it came as a surprise when he broke with tradition one morning and addressed me directly.

'OK, Mr Pringle, this is the situation. You and your colleague have been called to a hotel where an incident has occurred. Several 999 calls have been made, but the scene is confused. You are the first emergency vehicle to arrive and are immediately confronted by two men limping down the steps towards you. One is bleeding heavily from several wounds, and the other is clutching his chest looking very ill. What course of action do you take?'

On the face of it there wasn't much of a decision to make, but there had to be a catch. The trouble was that I couldn't see it.

'Well,' I said, 'I suppose my partner and I would split up and assess the two patients individually.'

'And then?'

'If they needed hospital treatment we would trans-port them.'

Gerald brought his fingertips up to his lower lip and looked at me from the corner of one eye. 'And that's it? That's all you would think of doing?'

'Yes,' I said, perplexed. 'I don't see there's much else we could do.'

'You don't see what else you could do.' He repeated my words with slow deliberation and looked round the class while I tried to think what I'd missed.

'I could call for a second ambulance if both the patients were in a serious condition,' I added in desperation.

'If that's really all you would do, Mr Pringle, then congratulations . . .'

I relaxed a little as he returned his gaze to the ceiling.

'. . . You've just contributed, in no small way, to the deaths of three men and a young woman.'

I gaped at him. 'How . . . I mean . . . you didn't mention anybody else. How on earth could I have contributed to—?'

Gerald raised a hand.

'To put it in a nutshell, you're guilty of neglect. There had been a gas explosion in the hotel basement and the water main was ruptured. The four unfortunate people I mentioned were trapped down there and drowned. They could have been saved if you had taken immediate action.'

The scenario was too preposterous for words and, if it had been anybody other than Gerald talking, I wouldn't have taken it seriously for a moment.

'How was I supposed to know all this?' I asked, and added with a touch of defiance, 'Who in their right mind would suspect people might be drowning in a hotel?'

'That is exactly the point.' Gerald was smiling now. 'As you were first on the scene it was your job to find out.' He paced slowly back and forth as he spoke. 'What I have just described actually happened some years ago. Spain, I think it was. The emergency services wasted precious time treating the walking wounded and when they got round to making a proper assessment of the situation it was too late for the people in the cellar.' Having set me up nicely as the fall guy, he stopped pacing and looked at the class. 'This is what we are going to spend the rest of the day examining: major incidents and our response to them.'

That night the dreams went a bit further. This time people were pulling at me from all sides as I fought to save the oxygen-starved butcher. They were shouting that a little girl was clinging on to the edge of a mine-shaft and I was the only person who could tie the knot that would pull her to safety. A rope was thrust at me but when I tried to take it I found my hands were moving through treacle. The girl was going to fall at any moment and I had to get the knot right at the first attempt, but I couldn't move my arms properly. Then Gerald was speaking to me.

'What about the people drowning in the cellar? Are you going to do anything about them, Mr Pringle?'

'I have to save the child, Gerald! Surely she comes first,' I gasped.

'It must be horrible in that cellar,' Gerald continued. 'Can you imagine it? And then there's the butcher, don't forget the butcher. He's turning blue, poor man. By the look of him he can't have more than a couple of minutes left.'

'I can't help them all! I can't even tie the knot!' I wailed.

'You are in charge, Mr Pringle. Everyone is depending on you, but you know that, don't you?'

The spell was broken when Gerald faded into the shadows, to be replaced by Roger offering me a piece of black pudding on a cocktail stick.

We celebrated the end of the course by holding a little party in the upstairs room of a local pub. It was a good night, despite being tinged with a little sadness. You get to know people quite well when you're all cooped up in an attic for six weeks, and a few real friendships had sprung up. We were delighted to have passed out but, on the other hand, it meant our group was about to be split up and scattered round different ambulance stations in the region. There was also the unspoken fear of stepping from the classroom into the real world.

At the end of the evening Mike and Gerald were given a silver Parker pen each as a gift from the group. Roger had been keen to make a little presentation speech and we found out why when he set about mimicking Gerald's deadpan delivery with wicked accuracy. Gerald joined in the laughter but, true to form, I don't think he really knew what the joke was.

Chapter Five

Henrietta Street Ambulance Station, more commonly known as 'the Street', sat squat and ugly amid a bleak landscape of post-war factories and warehouses close to Birmingham city centre. The run-down terraced houses of Lozells and Handsworth lay a mile away and even closer were Newtown and Aston, the epitome of inner-city deprivation. By way of light relief, three hostels for destitute alcoholics were only a short walk away. And as if that wasn't enough, the tough and uncompromising Street reputedly harboured all the rogue ambulance personnel in the West Midlands. A rumour going round, which I later found to be true, claimed someone had actually been transferred there as punishment for a misdemeanour. In short, we newcomers saw it as a place to be avoided at all costs, a penal colony where the life expectancy of a new recruit could be measured in days.

Plenty of other depots scattered around the region

needed replacement staff, so I didn't feel unduly apprehensive as I opened the letter. The sight of Gerald hovering close by wearing the face of a bereavement counsellor should have set off a few alarm bells, but I was on a roll, and confident the luck I'd enjoyed so far wouldn't desert me. I was wrong, of course. The words 'report to Henrietta Street' leaped from the page. In fact, they weren't content to leap from the page; they sprang up and grabbed me by the throat. Gerald had been waiting for his cue and, short of putting an arm round my shoulder, set about trying to convince me that it wasn't the end of the world. Not that I was listening.

After rereading the opening paragraph ten times in the hope I'd been mistaken, I discovered that I was joining 'C' shift, the very people who had rigged the handbrake for my driving test. I exhaled a long, slow breath and allowed Gerald's voice to drone back into focus. He was doing his best, but it didn't help much.

'. . . don't worry; it's not nearly as bad a place as they say it is. Just keep your head down and your mouth shut for the first few months and you'll be OK. You never know, you might be able to transfer out by the end of the year.'

My only consolation came when Roger, who'd been taking malicious delight in my discomfiture, opened his own letter and found he was joining me, albeit on a different shift.

I was to report the following Monday at 10 p.m. for the start of the night shift. This gave me the weekend to work myself into a state of near nervous collapse. It wasn't so much the thought of Henrietta Street, though heaven knows that was bad enough, it was more a case of old-fashioned cold feet. The more I fretted over what was to come, the more convinced I became that the whole idea had been a ghastly mistake from the start. Who did I think I was kidding? I'd none of the qualities needed to man an ambulance. Decisiveness and cool nerves were prerequisites, and there I was shaking like a leaf, barely able to make up my mind which side of the bed to get out of.

By the time I dragged myself into the messroom on that first night I knew I was an impostor just waiting to be found out. And my stretched nerves weren't eased by the frosty reception afforded me by the afternoon shift waiting to go home. It was a mistake to arrive well before my own shift came on duty, and I paid for it by being comprehensively ignored by everyone in the room. Left to wander around in my squeaky new uniform and feeling more self-conscious than I'd ever felt in my life, I took refuge in immersing myself in the standing orders pinned to the noticeboard. It did cross my mind to sit down and hide behind a newspaper, but I ruled it out for fear of picking a chair that might belong to one of the old hands.

It seemed an eternity before the members of 'C' shift started trooping through the door, but any relief I felt was quickly dampened when they greeted me with little more than sideways looks and guarded nods. I remained by the noticeboard like the new boy at school hoping to catch at least one friendly eye. Eventually, and somewhat reluctantly, it seemed to me, one of them uncoiled from his chair and came over. He was about thirty, six feet two and painfully thin. I caught a glimpse of tombstone teeth as his face contorted into something between a grimace and a smile.

'Hello, I'm Larry. It looks as though you're working with me this week.'

'Oh, hello, my name's Les Pri—'

'Yes, I know. Am I right in thinking you're straight out of training school?'

This was something I couldn't deny, especially as it was all but tattooed across my forehead.

He sighed and regarded me with the look of someone who'd just drawn Rotherham United in the office football sweep.

'Bloody great. Oh well, you might as well start by checking the truck and seeing if there's anything we need.'

Grateful for any excuse to escape, I was off into the garage like a shot.

You didn't need to be a sensitive soul to detect a lack of warmth in Larry's greeting. The essence of the matter was as true then as it is now: very few people like to work with new recruits. It's nothing personal. Given the choice of fussing round a newcomer like a mother hen, or having a relaxing day with someone you know and trust . . . well, it isn't really a choice at all. As a result, newbies are relentlessly batted between established shift members until some of the shine is worn off. In my case the batting had probably started days earlier, and Larry had come out the loser.

In no hurry to return to the messroom, I checked and rechecked the equipment; then leaned back in the attendant's seat to take a more leisurely view of my surroundings. Ambulances these days are designed with little else in mind but stark efficiency. It's not a surprising development, but it comes at the cost of losing some of the reassuring homeliness that patients used to find so comforting. The ambulance I was sitting in was smaller than its modern-day counterpart, the lighting softer, the colours warmer; it felt like being cocooned in the ultimate security blanket. Even the Automan with all its pipes and bellows sitting on the shelf opposite seemed to smile benignly, if you looked at it long enough. There was no doubt about it, I felt at home in this snug little world, and as I breathed in the odour of woollen blankets and freshly laundered linen I began to relax for the first time in days.

The sight of Larry suddenly appearing at the back doors with a mug of tea brought me out of my reverie with a start.

'Thought you might like a cup of tea, Les.' He placed it on the back step and retraced his steps before I had the wit to say thank you. I wouldn't have thought it possible that a cup of tea could raise my spirits as much as that one did. At first I didn't move, content to stare at the mug and savour its symbolic value. And the fact that Larry had personalized the gesture by using my name wasn't lost on me either. If I'd known it was to be the last cup of tea anyone would make me for the next eighteen months or so I would have appreciated it even more. As the rookie on the shift, tea-making was my job from then on.

I spent the rest of the night on a knife-edge. Amazingly, the others sat around playing Scrabble as if they hadn't a care in the world. I marvelled at their composure. My heart skipped a beat every time the phone rang, and sweat would break out on the palms of my hands to such a degree that I had to keep surreptitiously wiping it away on my trouser leg. While I tried desperately to remember how to tie a slipknot, or mentally worked my way through the resuscitation procedure, they were arguing about some obscure word on the Scrabble board. How did they stay so cool when at any moment a ring of the phone could plunge them into a drama of epic proportions? The answer was obvious. They were supermen.

As things worked out, and much to my relief, the cases we dealt with those first few nights could only be described as routine. Certainly not routine for the patients, of course, but for us there was little we could offer them but tender loving care. Children with high temperatures, the elderly with chest or bladder infections, all in all a catalogue of medical conditions the GPs considered worthy of following up in hospital. Even so, I hung on Larry's every action and word in a state of nervous agitation, which irritated me, never mind him. At best, he tolerated me. But he had an irreverent and cynical attitude to most things in life, to the point where I began to lose hope of ever getting a serious word out of him. The amazing thing was the way he changed when it came to patient care. In front of my eyes he metamorphosed into a tender, caring individual who was clearly in his element helping others. I can't imagine any patient looking on him as anything less than a saint. It was all very odd, but it was a trait I came to see in a lot of my colleagues over time.

It was on the fourth night I discovered that the only predictable aspect of the job is its unpredictability. Tackling imaginary scenarios in the comfort of the classroom had been one thing, getting to grips with the reality out on the road proved to be quite another. I know the instructors can't prepare you for everything, and I shouldn't really moan; it's just that they have a tendency to lull you into believing there's a logical answer to every problem. Everything is portrayed as black or white, never grey. The volunteer patients we practised on were always compliant, helpful even, leaving us students with the happy feeling that if we remembered all we were taught, then things would fall neatly into place. Well, if you ever read this, Gerald, I've got news for you. It doesn't always work that way.

And, what's more, it only took me four days to find out, courtesy of a gentleman called Michael.

Larry and I had been fruitlessly searching a dimly lit car park for someone with an injured leg when we picked up on a weird bellowing noise. We found a man furiously shadowboxing in front of a couple of wary-looking characters positioned just out of range of the flying fists. They didn't seem offended by the intermittent barrage of expletive-laden threats, but when Michael stopped bobbing and weaving to deliver a blistering flurry of combination punches they both took small but deliberate steps backwards. What I suspect kept them there was the imminent prospect of seeing Michael fall down; an event well overdue if the way he was lurching and staggering was anything to go by.

Above his waist everything was working like a well-oiled machine, but that couldn't be said for what was going on down below. His legs seemed to have a mind of their own. The right one was firmly rooted to the ground while the other thrashed madly this way and that. In the semi-darkness the errant limb gave the impression that it was trying to escape, but a closer look revealed that it was engaged in a battle to maintain Michael's constantly shifting balance. Not that Michael seemed aware of the fight going on to keep him upright; he blithely boxed on while hurling abuse at anyone who caught his eye. Larry and I watched the manic display in silence, neither of us wanting to admit that we had probably found our patient.

It was gone eleven o'clock and the pub opposite was slowly disgorging the last of its clientele, who, attracted by the commotion, drifted over in twos and threes to watch. Soon a fair few people were jostling for position, and it wasn't long before one of them felt compelled to come over for a friendly word.

'Come for Michael, have you? I've got to hand it to you blokes, you gotta have some balls to do your job, so you have.'

As an accolade, it was unsettling.

'What do you mean?'

He leaned towards me.

'I mean, Michael's an awful man when he's got the drink in him! I've seen him take apart men twice your size.'

He smelled as if he'd just climbed out of a Guinness barrel but I held my ground in the hope of hearing something constructive.

'Sounds like you know him then.'

'Know him!' He gave me a second look to check I was being serious. 'Everybody knows him. It's Michael Neil you're looking at!' He dropped this intended bombshell with a mixture of awe and relish, and waited for the reaction. When he didn't get one, he looked incredulous. 'Surely you've run into him before?'

'No, I don't think I have,' I said, not wanting to reveal that this was only my fourth day in the job.

'Really? Well, you're in for a treat. It's the same

every weekend, he gets pissed, and then he starts fighting. By the end of the night he's either in nick or in hospital. Mind you, when the police come for him they're usually mob-handed.'

Not gleaning much comfort from these words, I looked back at Michael to find him throwing a sequence of lightning-fast rabbit punches while emitting professional-sounding snorts and sniffs. He wasn't a particularly big man, I would say about five foot nine and probably in his early forties, but his hands were like shovels, and he had that wiry, mean look of a street fighter. There wasn't any doubt in my mind that a tactical retreat was called for but it was already too late; Michael caught sight of our uniforms and, with his face contorted in fury, redirected his shouts at us.

'Hey! You two! Have you ever been punched by an Irishman?' He glared at us and threw a demonstration punch into the air. 'Well? I asked you a fuck'n' question! Have you ever been punched by an Irishman?'

To my consternation, Larry shouted back, 'Of course we have . . . who hasn't been?'

Michael's eyes narrowed and he stopped boxing for a moment.

'Oh, so we're a smartarse, are we? I'm warning you . . . you lanky arsehole . . . clear off now, and take your fuck'n' ambulance with you . . . unless you want to have it rammed up your arse!'

I was gobsmacked. Despite many warnings that

manning an inner-city ambulance wasn't going to be a bed of roses, deep down I still believed most of my time would be spent mopping fevered brows while whispering words of reassurance into grateful ears. The possibility of being threatened and sworn at hadn't crossed my mind. Out of my depth, and feeling distinctly uncomfortable, I looked back at Larry to see how he was going to handle things. To my surprise he was standing with his hands in his pockets, smiling.

'Do you think we should call for the police?' I asked when it became clear he wasn't going to say anything.

'The police! You must be joking. It's Friday night; they wouldn't turn up for hours. Besides, we don't even know if he's our patient.'

This was true, but it seemed likely he was. We were looking for a man with a leg injury and, judging by Michael's strangely immobile limb, there was every chance it was him.

'So,' I asked tentatively, 'what are we going to do?'

Larry took his eyes off Michael and looked at me with a pained expression. 'You're the attendant; it's up to you where we go from here.'

Putting new recruits on the spot isn't just an effective way of bringing home to them how helpless they are without guidance, it reaffirms, if they need it reaffirming, exactly where they stand in the pecking order. On this occasion Larry had the added bonus of having a bit of fun at my expense. I pondered the situation and came to the conclusion that I didn't have a clue what to do next.

'To be honest, Larry, I can't quite see where to go from here. He doesn't seem to like us very much and—'

'You've just come out of training school, haven't you? Who was your tutor?'

'Gerald Hastings,' I said, surprised by the defensive tone in my voice.

Larry threw back his head and laughed. 'There you go then! You should have all the answers. Just think back and try to imagine how Gerald would have handled it.'

I was thinking, and getting nowhere. 'We didn't actually cover this kind of scenario,' I eventually bleated.

'OK, I'll give you a clue. Start by talking to the bloke.' Larry was enjoying himself all right. 'See if you can build up a relationship of mutual trust and understanding. Go on.'

Despite not relishing the idea of getting any closer to Michael than I had to, I edged forward gingerly.

'Hello, Michael. What's wrong with your leg, have you hurt it?'

'I've told you once . . . piss off!'

This was the best advice I'd had so far but before I acted on it I had to at least establish if he really was our patient.

'We only want to help you. Be reasonable. If you're OK we'll go.'

'You're starting to get on my tits . . . Clear off out of here, you slimy git!'

'There's no need to be like—'

'Piss off!'

I wasn't to know it at the time, but this was the first futile conversation in what was to be a long career of futile conversations. I still find them rather trying. I mean, what on earth do you say next? How do you placate someone who has no desire to be placated? I was groping for my next line when at last Larry intervened.

'Come on, let's go, I'm fed up of this. I don't see why we should hang around here and risk getting our heads punched . . .'

He broke off in mid-sentence. A passing car's head-lights had momentarily illuminated the swaying Irishman and, in that instant, it became horribly clear that Michael was our patient and, more to the point, whether he liked it or not he was going to end up in the back of our ambulance.

He had a fractured ankle. But it wasn't just any old fracture; it was grotesque. His foot was splayed out at right angles to the leg, with the stump taking most of his weight. The good leg, which was constantly flapping around to maintain his balance, made his whole body rotate slowly on exposed bone. It looked excruciatingly painful and the sight made all of us watching feel slightly sick. Leaving him to his own devices was out of the question: one way or the other he had to go to hospital. Cautiously, I moved in even closer while pleading with him.

'Michael, just look at your foot. It's going to fall off, for Christ's sake.'

'I've warned you! As God's my witness, so help me, I've warned you! Come any closer and you'll get a taste of this!' He threw a punch into the air that almost toppled him over.

It was a ludicrous stand-off and, for good measure, the now-sizeable group of drinkers gathered round began to make matters worse. They were delighted by the after-hours entertainment we were laying on, some even taking malicious pleasure in winding Michael up further by shouting encouragement and advice.

'You tell 'em, Mick, don't you stand for it. Knock their bloody heads off if they try anything!'

Others took a less light-hearted view, and rounded on us indignantly. 'What's wrong with you two? Can't you see the poor man's injured? You should be doing something!'

Again I felt hot, beer-laden breath wafting over me.

'Do you want me to knock him out for you?'

'What?'

'Just give the word and I'll knock him out.'

I couldn't quite believe what I was hearing.

'Knock him out? Are you out of your skull? We're not here to mug him, for Christ's sake!'

He wasn't listening though.

'I could do it for you! One good pisser on the

jaw would be enough; it would be like an act of mercy, wouldn't it? You know what I mean, like an act of God sent to put him out of his misery, so to speak.'

He had a glint in his eye that made me think his enthusiasm for the task wasn't altogether altruistic.

'You can't be serious! Do you want us all to end up in a police cell for the night?' I tried to think of a way round the problem. 'Hasn't he got any friends here that can reason with him?'

The man grinned. 'Believe me, when he's sober he's everybody's friend, but when he's pissed he's a real nasty piece of work. Everybody gives him a very wide berth. Oh, and another thing . . . I better warn you that he never forgets a face. If you upset him you'd do well not to show up round here again in a hurry.'

'Well, thanks for that. You aren't helping much, are you?' I looked back at Michael, who, like a poor man's Long John Silver, stood grinning inanely at the crowd. Their shouts of encouragement spurred him on, while the couple of gallons of beer fermenting in his belly had rendered him oblivious to the pain.

Larry pulled me aside to talk things through. The ideal solution was obvious: bring him down with a tranquillizer dart, throw a net over him and then, using the crowd as bearers, carry him off to hospital on a pole. If only things were that simple. Contrary to what most people assume, we have no power to force anyone into the ambulance against their will. It would be tantamount to kidnap. If the patient is unconscious there isn't a problem, but if he's awake then it's his inalienable right to tell whomever it is trying to help him to get lost. (Unless he's 'sectioned', of course. Then, under the Mental Health Act, the state can take complete control of his life and only give it back to him when it sees fit.) As things stood, even to lay a hand on him without his consent could be classed as assault. After considering all the legal ramifications, Larry came to a decision. We would deny him his human rights, assault him, and then kidnap him for good measure.

We would need help. It wasn't easy finding three sober enough people from the crowd, but when we eventually had them on board Larry gathered us together and set out his plan of attack with military precision:

1. The three helpers would position themselves behind the patient while Larry and I distracted him from the front.
2. On command, the helpers would rush Michael and bring him to the ground.
3. I would grab the damaged limb and hold it steady.
4. Larry would fix the splint in position.
5. We would then throw him in the ambulance.

The helpers were grinning. The way they seemed to relish the whole idea made me slightly uneasy, but what the heck, I didn't see that we had much choice. As we all moved into position I thought back to training school. Try as I might, I couldn't remember getting any advice from Gerald on the best way to attack a patient.

'Michael!' Larry shouted out. 'We're coming to get you!'

Michael looked amused at the idea and, raising his fists in preparation, shouted back, 'Is that a fact? Well, come on then, you lanky fucker.'

'*Go!*' Larry gave the command before he got any further.

Michael, taken by surprise by an attack from the rear, went down in a flurry of limbs. The onlookers cheered and shouted advice as he struggled, but he was soon overpowered. A moment later I had the damaged leg firmly in my grasp as Larry manoeuvred the dangling foot into position and secured it in the splint. Michael, realizing the game was up, stopped resisting and restricted himself to pouring out an unrelenting stream of obscenities. Defeated but unbowed, he allowed himself to be lifted into the ambulance while acknowledging the cheering crowd with a smile and a regal wave.

'It wasn't a fair fight!' he bellowed at them. 'You all saw it . . . five against one! It took five of the fuckers! Next time it'll be better odds. Do you hear what I'm saying, it wasn't a fair fight, five against—'

His ranting was cut short when I slammed the back doors on him. Shutting the doors was like bringing the curtain down on what, I have to admit, was a pretty impressive performance, a performance that wouldn't do his reputation in these parts any harm at all.

Chapter Six

Mike Andrews was our shift leader. It wasn't an official position, more a statement of fact. Weighing in at somewhere near eighteen stone, and just over six feet tall, he tended to get noticed. But it wasn't just his appearance that shaped people's reaction to him; the strength of his personality alone commanded immediate respect. He was well into his fifties when I joined the shift and it was immediately noticeable how others not much his junior deferred to him without question. As for the likes of me, well, just to be on the receiving end of a raised eyebrow was enough to stop me in my tracks. No doubt the years he'd spent as a sergeant in the Marines helped mould him, but that wouldn't explain the very real affection in which he was held. Anyone working with him soon came to realize that under the irascible, disapproving father figure lay a man of genuine compassion and warmth.

He had his faults of course, plenty of them. The

worst, in my opinion, was the self-delusion that he was something of a chef. It was a tradition on the shift to cook a meal at work occasionally; usually at about 1 a.m. when things had quietened down a bit. Everyone had their own speciality and we would take turns to cook something simple like spaghetti bolognaise or curry. Mike set his sights higher. When his turn came round, and no matter how hard the ingredients were to come by, he would serve us one of the devilish recipes he'd picked up in his military days. The one I came to dread most was a chilli-based South American dish. He would ladle it on to our plates with huge chunks of bread hacked from a loaf. The idea behind the bread, I quickly found out, was to stuff it into your mouth after a spoonful of chilli in the hope of diffusing some of the heat.

While we struggled, Mike would sit at the head of the table like a brooding Buddha. Ignoring the regular interruptions of hiccups, sneezing and the blowing of noses, he would become misty-eyed as he described adventures from his army days in obscure parts of the world. We would sit drenched in sweat, listening to how he spent a week hiding in a swamp to ambush local insurgents somewhere in Malaya. Much of the time, he would have us believe, was spent under water breathing through a snorkel with a jungle knife at the ready. When night fell, he and his comrades would emerge from the swamp and eat from a menu consisting of anything that happened to crawl or slither past.

Such memories would inspire him to list many other hardships he'd endured, and inform the younger ones at the table that we didn't know we'd been born. If we were unaware of it before sitting down to the meal, we certainly knew it after a mouthful of chilli. We kept a wary eye on one another, each fearful that he would be the first to falter. Eventually, someone would splutter and push away their plate, saying that it was the best chilli he'd ever tasted but he couldn't manage any more. This would bring down Mike's scorn on his head.

'You've hardly touched it! What are you, a man or a mouse? Where's your backbone? You wouldn't last two minutes in the real world!' Then, to the horror of the rest of us, he would share out our mate's unwanted food on to our plates.

Of course, I wasn't to know any of this when Larry casually mentioned that Mike would be cooking us a meal on Sunday night. In my ignorance, I was pleased by the prospect of sitting round the table with the rest of the shift and maybe getting to know them a little better. When the big night arrived, Mike's ambulance went to the back of the running order and he spent three quarters of an hour whistling and humming to himself as he stirred the bubbling cauldron, stopping occasionally to add a pinch of this or that. The smell coming from the kitchen was heavenly, and by the time we took up position at the table my mouth was watering in anticipation. A subdued atmosphere seemed to have descended on the room but I put it down to my imagination and scooped a hefty spoonful of the chilli stew into my mouth. Hot food was nothing new to me, and I wouldn't have put myself down as a softie, but this was something else altogether. It was like biting into a nest of scorpions. My eyes and nose watered instantly, and if tongues can writhe in pain, then mine writhed.

When my vision cleared I looked up to find I was being watched intently. Mike's jaws were working hard while the others sat with a hunk of bread in one hand and very small portions of chilli on the end of their spoons, which they didn't seem in any hurry to eat. Larry was smiling, while Howard, a chap I'd already put down as one of the more kindly shift members, proffered me his bread. I crammed it into my mouth just as the emergency phone rang.

Larry dragged his eyes off me and, clanking his spoon down in apparent frustration, swore loudly.

'Isn't that just typical! How do they always manage to ring that bloody phone at the exact moment we sit down to eat?' He looked over at Mike. 'Sorry, Mike, it was one of your better ones as well.'

Mike gazed at him suspiciously from behind a spoonful of chilli. 'It'll still be here when you get back.'

Larry gave a nervous laugh. 'It had better be.'

'It will be,' Mike assured him.

There was a spring in Larry's step as we walked out to the ambulance.

'Talk about being saved by the bell! I was praying we'd get a job and then, bingo! The phone rings. What did you think of Mike's molten lava? Good stuff, eh?'

I was determined not to let him see I was still in pain and tried a bit of irony.

'Oh, very nice. A little on the hot side perhaps.' Then, sounding as casual as I could, I asked, 'So what's this job we're going to?'

Larry wasn't ready to be diverted from the chilli. 'A little on the hot side! You need an asbestos mouth to eat one of Mike's concoctions. He might have lost his own taste buds thirty years ago, but I want to hang on to mine.'

'Yes, I see your point. So, er, what's wrong with our patient?'

'Oh yes, the patient: it's a woman having difficulty breathing.'

My mind went into immediate overdrive as I climbed into the attendant's seat.

'Might it be something like asthma?'

'That's possible,' Larry answered laconically. 'Of course it might just as easily be heart failure. That causes the lungs to fill up with fluid and affects the breathing – very nasty.'

I gulped.

'Then again,' he continued, 'she might be having an allergic reaction. Her tongue could be swelling up and cutting off her air supply.'

I rubbed the palms of my hands against my trouser legs.

'And you can't discount trauma,' Larry added brightly as he swung the ambulance on to the main road. 'She might have had some kind of accident and have a collapsed lung, two even. If she's been stabbed, then we're looking at a pneumothorax.'

'Stabbed!' I almost squeaked.

He took his eye off the road for a moment and addressed me in a worryingly serious tone.

'Look, when we get there just leave everything to me, and stay close in case I need you. Got that?'

'Yes, got it.'

Larry returned his attention to the road. 'That's the thing about this life . . . you never really know what's coming your way. You have to be prepared for virtually anything.'

I reached behind the seat and pulled the oxygen bag on to my lap.

By the time we drew up in front of the small terraced house there was so much adrenalin thumping round my system that I was scrabbling for the door handle before the ambulance came to a halt.

'Hey! Calm down.' Larry sounded almost alarmed. 'I'm to go in first, remember?'

As the attendant, it was really my job to make first contact with the patient, but I was grateful to bring up the rear as Larry picked his way down a path crowded by a jungle of overgrown shrubs and knee-high grass.

He rang the bell and then nonchalantly leaned against the wall, picking at a strip of paint flaking from the door. I would never be that cool; if I stayed on the job for a hundred years, I would never be that cool.

Half a minute later the hall light went on and the tremulous voice of an elderly lady came from inside.

'Who is it?'

'It's the ambulance service.'

The door opened a couple of inches and Larry leaned forward to speak into the gap.

'Hello, Mary, how are you tonight?'

'I'm very well, thank you. How are you?'

'Oh, I'm fine,' Larry said. 'Can I come in?'

'Of course you can, my love, and bring your friend too.'

Bemused and still clutching the oxygen bag, I followed Larry into the house.

She couldn't have weighed more than six stone and must have been at least ninety. Her arthritic hand reached out and clutched Larry's sleeve for support as she squinted up into his face.

'You're the nice young man who came to see me last week, aren't you?'

'That's right, Mary, and the week before. What's the matter tonight?'

'Well, nothing worth talking about really. I'm just being silly as usual. Would you and your friend like a nice cup of tea?'

Larry smiled. 'That's probably the best offer we'll get all night.'

She gave him an impish grin and was turning in the direction of the kitchen when he reached out and gently caught her by the arm.

'Whoa, hold your horses. Les will make the tea, he needs the practice. Why don't we sit down in the living room and have a chat while he gets on with it.'

Larry looked at me over her head and winked before nodding towards the kitchen.

I put down the oxygen with a petulant thump that I hoped wouldn't go unnoticed and went through to the kitchen knowing I'd been done up like a kipper. Clearly, Larry knew exactly what to expect when he read the address on the case sheet and, true to form, had grabbed the opportunity to have a little fun at my expense.

I filled the kettle and listened to them chatting while it boiled. She was doing most of the talking with Larry encouraging her by dropping in the odd interjection. As far as I could make out, the topic was her life as a factory girl during the First World War. She was describing, amid laughter, the monstrous men's overalls she was forced to wear when I brought in the pot of tea and placed it on a small table by her chair. I then returned for the milk, sugar and cups and watched anxiously as she insisted on pouring even though she barely had the strength to lift the pot.

'Where are the biscuits?' She looked about her. 'You've forgotten the biscuits.'

'Sorry, I didn't realize . . .'

'There are some nice ginger snaps in the cupboard. You wait here and I'll fetch them.'

The moment she left the room I leaned over and hissed at Larry. 'She doesn't look like someone having difficulty breathing to me. What's supposed to be wrong with her?'

'She's old and a bit confused, that's all.'

'That's it?'

'That's it,' Larry repeated.

I exhaled slowly to show my exasperation. 'I can't believe you wound me up like that and then sent me off to make a pot of tea.'

'Didn't Gerald get you to play out the tea-making scenario?'

'No! It must have slipped his mind.'

Larry smiled. 'A cup of tea and a chat is all the treatment she needs. She's fine during the day, but sometimes she wakes up at night frightened. It could be anything that spooks her, a cat going through the bins, or maybe just the wind in the trees. Whatever it is, she gets the night terrors and ends up ringing us saying she can't breathe properly.' He took a sip of tea. 'The trick is to get her to talk about something that will take her mind off whatever's upset her, usually something from the past. She soon calms down and eventually goes back to bed without a care in the world.'

'But is this kind of thing really our job?' I asked, keeping my voice low.

'Of course it's our job!' Larry said. 'Whose job do you think it is? If we go out to the likes of Michael threatening to punch our heads in, then we can damn well spend a little time on someone like Mary. If she was your grandmother, how would you want her to be treated?' He took another sip of tea and grimaced. 'God, you're going to have to improve.'

Ten minutes later Mary was ushering us down the hall insisting that we should call again soon. Larry opened the door and was turning to wish her good night when she let out a little cry of surprise and pointed out into the street.

'Oh look! There's an ambulance outside. I do hope nobody's been hurt.'

Back in the cab Larry looked at his watch in annoyance.

'We've only been out for half an hour, damn it. Our best hope is to get another job or we'll be staring at Mike's bloody chilli again.'

As if in answer to his plea, Control obliged by straight away giving us another 999. Larry happily wrote down the details, until it came to the address.

'God! I'd rather face the chilli!'

'Why?' I asked. 'What's the problem?'

'We're going to "an unwell man" at the Sundown Centre. You won't have heard of the place unless you've got a secret past. It's a dosshouse for homeless alcoholics. It's the pits . . . a dump.'

The first thing to hit you on entering a hostel for

alcoholics is the unique smell oozing from the fabric of the building. The constituents are simple: cider, cigarette smoke, body odour and unwashed clothes. Mix them in roughly equal quantities, add a total lack of ventilation and you will more or less have it.

We kept our breathing as shallow as possible as the night warden led us up to one of the rooms on the third floor. He couldn't have been more than forty but he had the air of someone who'd been battered and ultimately defeated by life a long time ago. A cigarette was cupped in his left hand and swaying from his right was a large bunch of keys, the weight of which seemed almost too much for him. We trailed the thin, hunched figure through a maze of corridors trying not to listen as he grumbled about the residents in his charge. If he was to be believed, and he had us convinced, the only reason they'd been put on this earth was to make his life unbearable. Eventually he stopped at one of the rooms and inserted a key in the lock.

With the opening of the door, a rush of hot, fetid air escaped on to the landing. We took an involuntary step backwards and squinted through the thinning fug of cigarette smoke. It was a small, cramped room containing a bed, armchair, washbasin and coffee table. Three men were sitting on the floor round the table and behind them another man was slumped in the armchair. Playing cards were spread out over the table along with a few coins and glasses of cider. The three men, befuddled by drink, put their cards down and stared at us. They had nothing to say and seemed to be trying to work out who we were. The warden, on the other hand, had plenty to say. He erupted in anger at the vacant faces.

'You're drinking! You're drinking in the building! You know it's not allowed. You'll all be on the street tomorrow . . . and that's a promise!' His lower lip trembled and he waited for his words to sink home before dragging himself back to the matter in hand.

'Well! You wanted an ambulance! Come on then, these men are busy, which one of you is supposed to be ill?' This didn't bring an immediate response, so he fixed the nearest man with a withering glare. 'Spit it out, man. What's the problem?'

'Ah . . . yes! It's Jimmy.' The man waved an arm towards the figure in the armchair. 'He's not well. He just wants to sleep and won't even finish his drink. I poured that one for him more than an hour ago and he hasn't touched it.' He pointed at a full glass sitting at the man's feet. Before he could continue the warden broke in.

'You're not telling me you've called these men out in the middle of the night because Jimmy here won't drink his cider!'

The man slowly assembled his thoughts. 'No, course not. He's not well. Take a look at him for yourself.'

While they were talking I had been looking at the man in the chair. From five feet away, and even with my lack of experience, it was obvious he was dead.

Larry squeezed past the table and searched in vain for a pulse while taking a closer look at the patient. His lips were a deep purple set in a pasty white face; he must have been dead for quite some time. Larry straightened up and turned to the others.

'I'm sorry, we can't help him.'

One of the men sitting on the floor put down his hand of cards and spoke up indignantly. 'What do you mean you can't help him? You've got to! You don't have to be a doctor to see he's not well!'

His companion lurched to his feet and took a couple of drunken steps towards the dead man. After some deliberation he came to much the same conclusion as his friend.

'He doesn't look very well to me either. Don't get me wrong, I'm not a medical man, you understand, but I think my mate's right. He needs to go to hospital and get sorted.'

Larry and I looked at each other; this clearly wasn't the time or place for subtleties.

'We can't help him because he's dead!' To give his words some extra weight Larry stared at each of them in turn. 'And, what's more, he's been dead for ages.'

This was met by silence, then a smile slowly spread over the 'non-medical' man's face. It struck me that he might think Larry was making a macabre joke.

'Look, my friend's right,' I said. 'He's dead. We can't do anything.'

This time the message got through, but the first person to find his voice was the warden.

'You . . . you . . . you stupid bastards! You've been sitting here all night playing cards with a corpse and you didn't even notice! In the name of God . . . !'

One of the men lurched over to the body and threw his arms round it. He held it for a moment, and then started to wail. 'Jimmy, Jimmy, wake up! You can't be dead . . . Jimmy!'

There was an awkward pause while we watched him pour out his grief, but we had to move on. We needed to gather a few details about the patient, and started by asking for his full name. The occupants of the room looked at each other and when it became obvious that none of them knew, the warden could barely contain himself.

'Come on, come on. You know his first name's Jimmy, what's his second name?'

'I call everybody Jimmy,' said the man with his arms round the body.

The warden stared at him for a full two seconds. 'You can't be seriously telling me that you don't even know him!' His gimlet eye then ranged over the rest of them. 'What's his bloody room number then?'

No reply, and the tiny bit of patience the warden had left evaporated. 'Come on, one of you must know!'

The man supporting the body disengaged himself and, looking decidedly ill at ease, spoke up. 'Strictly speaking, he's not actually stopping here. We met him at the coach station.'

'You met him at the coach station?' The warden mouthed the words back at him before exploding. 'You *know* non-residents aren't allowed in the rooms! There are notices all over the fucking building!' Then he added, a little unnecessarily, I thought, 'Especially fucking dead ones! What am I going to do with him? Go on . . . tell me! Tell me what I'm supposed to do with a corpse without a name in the middle of the night? Take him home and put him in my fucking spare room?'

If he was expecting any suggestions from the men he was disappointed. They avoided his gaze and, in doing so, one of them noticed the untouched glass of cider at Jimmy's feet. He leaned forward and picked it up and, raising it to his lips, said, 'Well, he won't be wanting this now, will he?' and drained it in one go.

Chapter Seven

There was just the hint of a smile on Larry's face as he passed over the allocation sheet.

'Well, well. Looks like you're working with Mike tomorrow.'

I nervously read down the list, hoping this was just another leg-pull. When I found my name next to Mike's I came near to having a seizure.

'God, he'll eat me alive!'

Larry stood up and stretched. 'I've a feeling you might be right. There's not much he can't eat. Just try not to upset him, especially in the morning.'

Job done, he wandered off whistling tunelessly to himself, leaving me with something new to brood over. Mike was the shift patriarch, and a particularly fearsome one at that. Inheriting the tiresome job of knocking me into shape wasn't likely to improve his demeanour one little bit.

Anxious not to wake anybody, I crept into the

messroom the next morning. To my surprise, Mike was already ensconced in his chair with a newspaper draped over his head. Heeding Larry's warning that he wasn't a man to be trifled with this early in the day, I tiptoed through to the kitchen and put the kettle on. The question now was whether to wake him with a cup of tea or let him sleep. I was still agonizing over what to do when a grunt emanated from behind the newspaper.

'Nobody made the tea yet?'

The words were hardly out of his mouth when I placed the mug on the armrest of his chair. 'There you are, Mike. Two sugars, isn't it?'

He pulled the newspaper away and sat up, rubbing his eyes. I watched over him like a fawning wine waiter as he took a sip.

'OK?'

'Fine.' He looked up at me as if wondering why I was still there. 'Have you checked everything's all right on the truck?'

'Well, no. I thought I'd make a brew and then do it.'

He took another sip of tea. 'Always check the truck first. You don't want to get into bad habits.'

The fact that no one at the Street had seen him check a vehicle in the last twenty years didn't seem to prick his conscience. But then with people like me around, why should it?

Several pots of tea later and I was getting edgy. We'd been on duty for over an hour and other than the occasional rustle of a newspaper, tranquillity reigned.

At least it reigned for the others. The longer I waited for a job to come through, the more nervous I became. I was glancing at the phone for what must have been the fiftieth time when it erupted into life with a squawk that had me on my feet more effectively than a cattle prod. I was only vaguely aware of the ironic cheer that went up from the others as I covered the three feet to the phone and snatched it up. Larry began talking loudly from his chair as I wrote down the case details.

'Someone better tell *The Guinness Book of Records*. That's got to be the fastest time ever for answering a phone.'

'Nah, remember Johnny Morris?' someone else said. 'He could have beaten that, no problem. If I remember rightly, he had a heart attack in the end.'

'No, you're thinking of Malcolm Tomlinson. In his prime Malcolm could make the phone in under two seconds from a sitting start.'

My face burned hot as I scurried out to the garage leaving the mock debate in full flight.

Mike was already behind the wheel.

'So, what have we got?'

I could have repeated the control girl's words verbatim but, determined to show a little more sangfroid, I pretended to read from the case sheet.

'Er, let me see . . . it's a woman collapsed in a car at the Brasshouse Centre off Broad Street.'

Mike smiled as he eased the ambulance out into the rush-hour traffic. 'The Brasshouse it is then.'

The old adage 'there's nowt stranger than folk' had already gained a certain resonance in my mind. Our training had focused on the diagnostic and practical side of things and little attention had been given to another, rather significant aspect of the job ... the foibles of human nature. If meeting Michael in the pub car park had come as an early warning shot across my bows, then the lady we were rushing to assist was about to fire the second salvo, albeit from a different angle. She fell into the surprisingly large group of people who, with very little effort, can turn a minor incident into a major catastrophe. But first we have to picture the scene leading up to the 999 call.

It was eight thirty on an overcast morning when the gleaming Jaguar entered the car park and swung into its reserved space in front of the office block. At the wheel sits an elegant woman in her early thirties, dressed expensively but severely in a dark two-piece business suit. Her hair is tied back and what make-up she's wearing has been applied sparingly and carefully. She exudes the air of effortless self-confidence and authority that comes with success. Just a glimpse is enough to tell anyone she's a person with her life well under control, someone who is more than capable of meeting any challenge the day might put her way.

She steps from the car, opens one of the rear doors and leans in to retrieve her briefcase, unconcerned that her skirt has ridden up a few inches to reveal a fair measure of thigh. As luck would have it, it's not a fortunate passer-by who notices; she's spotted by a torpid wasp that should have been in hibernation weeks earlier. For reasons only the wasp could explain, it swoops down to deliver a sting on one of the evenly tanned limbs.

If wasps take a perverse pleasure in stinging people, then this one must have been in its element as it savoured the resulting scream. To the other people arriving for work it probably sounded as if someone was being murdered, and they came running in panic from all corners of the car park to find her sprawled across the back seat of the car, her face buried in the soft leather upholstery, both hands clutching her leg. Listening to her muffled sobs, the would-be rescuers were unsure what to do. They had no idea what had happened, and their nervous enquiries didn't get them anywhere. Left with little choice, several of them ran off to find a telephone. As a result, Control received two or three garbled 999 calls.

We arrived to find the woman hyperventilating in the back of her car. Her eyes bulged and her chest heaved as she sucked in air as if each breath was to be her last. I hadn't seen anybody in the throws of a major panic attack before and, despite having covered it in training, I failed to recognize the problem when it was staring me in the face. All I could think of doing was to get her on oxygen as quickly as possible and ask questions later. Mike, of course, had other ideas. As I reached for the bag, he pushed it aside with his foot and leaned forward to address the woman in an unexpectedly firm voice.

'Madam! Will you please get yourself under control and explain what the problem is.'

His tone took both the woman and me by surprise. She looked up for the first time and with a shaking finger pointed feebly at her leg.

'I think . . . I think I've been stung.'

A quick glance revealed a red circle about the size of a five-pence coin just above the knee. Mike looked puzzled, and then indignant.

'Is that it? Is that what all the fuss is about?'

Still breathing as if she'd just staggered over the finish line of a marathon, she panted a few more words. 'It's all right for you. You're not . . . you're not . . . the one who's been stung.'

Mike raised his eyes skyward and seemed to be counting to ten under his breath.

It wasn't going to be easy to persuade the woman to slow her breathing but Mike composed himself and set about the task, using a subtle blend of reassurance and cajolement. I was watching the process keenly in the hope of learning something when one of the bystanders felt moved to offer me a piece of advice.

'I think she's in anti-phallic shock.'

'What?'

'Don't get me wrong, I'm not trying to tell you your job, but I think you should consider anti-phallic shock.'

I tried not to smile. 'Anaphylactic shock?'

'That's it! When someone's neck swells up and they can't breathe.'

Ever since the devastating effects of anaphylactic shock were highlighted on television, it has seemed that half the population believe they have only minutes left to live if a bee or wasp gives them so much as a sideways glance. The truth is that it's a very rare phenomenon. I've only seen it once in my entire career as the direct result of a sting. There was no mistaking it; it scared me half to death, never mind the patient.

Mike's perseverance bore fruit when the woman began to regain a semblance of self-control and accept her world wasn't about to come to an end. Her breathing rate returned to near normal levels, but not even Mike could convince her that her day wasn't ruined. Going into the office was out of the question and our last act of assistance was to guide her into one of her co-workers' cars. As we watched it pull out into the traffic with its white-faced passenger, Mike shook his head and said to no one in particular, 'She wouldn't last five minutes in the real world.'

He often referred to 'the real world' as if it were some mythical place only he'd been privileged to glimpse. If there is a 'real world' out there somewhere, and I'm not sure there is, then it begs the question . . . who lives in it? Certainly not the three unforgettable people Mike and I ran into the following week. They inhabited a little world of their own in the heart of a drab council estate just north of the city centre. They were the very antithesis of the woman stung by the wasp. When faced with a situation that would have any normal person screaming from the rooftops, this trio looked on the calamity that befell them as little more than a minor annoyance.

The details of the case were sketchy. It was passed to us as 'man bleeding'. It was six thirty in the morning, a bit early for people to start hurting themselves, so it seemed more likely to be a medical emergency, perhaps a bleeding ulcer or a burst varicose vein.

A hint of red streaked the horizon and the dawn chorus was tentatively starting up in the trees as we stepped from the ambulance. Not that we had long to savour this little moment of serenity: our mood was abruptly broken by the sight of a heavy-set, sullen-looking woman waiting on the doorstep. She wore a tatty dressing gown and was leaning heavily against the doorframe with the undisguised look of someone dragged from their sleep. She heaved her bulk away from the door with an air of supreme world-weariness and took a drag of her cigarette.

'He's upstairs in bed,' she said.

Mike's smile of greeting was effectively wiped from his face and, not being in the mood to try and win new friends, he deliberately adopted her blunt manner.

'Which bedroom?'

She took another pull on her cigarette and replied through the smoke. 'Front.'

The pleasantries over, the three of us made our way upstairs.

The small room was dominated by a large double bed harbouring a middle-aged man. He lay on his back staring at the ceiling and, curiously, didn't take the slightest interest in our arrival. The woman took up position near the window and stood staring out, her arms folded, the smoke from her cigarette drifting upwards. I waited for one of them to speak but when it became clear that neither was going to volunteer anything I turned my attention to the man in the bed. He looked pale and generally unwell. Clearly something was amiss, so I crouched down, introduced myself and asked his name.

'Tony.'

In uttering just one word, he managed to convey a degree of petulance that rankled with me even more than his failure to turn his head in my direction. None the less, I continued patiently. 'I'm told you're bleeding. What's happened?' Not getting a reply, I added a bit of edge to my voice. 'Tony, we're not here for our own good, you know. If you're bleeding, tell me about it.'

I took his pulse as I spoke. It was a bit fast but not too bad.

'It stopped bleeding ages ago,' Tony said, without taking his eyes off the ceiling.

'OK,' I said patiently. 'Where was the blood coming from?'

The woman flicked her fag out of the window and, acting like someone who'd finally lost patience with a naughty child, spoke in a voice heavy with sarcasm.

'Where from? He's got a knife sticking out of him and you ask where he's bleeding from! Where do you think he's bleeding from?'

'Knife?' I was mystified. 'What knife? Where?'

'*What knife?*' she repeated. 'Try the one in his neck for starters!' She moved closer, leaving a trail of last night's alcohol. 'How many do you think there are?'

Gingerly, I leaned over and peered at the side of Tony's neck so far hidden from me, and there it was . . . a small kitchen knife buried up to the hilt about an inch below the ear lobe. A path of dried brown blood snaked down into the sheets where it had gathered in a small crusty pool. I stared at the knife as if in a dream. If we'd been called to a pub fight, or an attack in the street, then I would have been prepared for a stabbing, but to be examining someone with a knife wound in their own bed at this time in the morning couldn't have come as more of a shock.

Judging by the handle, I estimated the blade to be something in the region of two and a half inches long. Tony had steady, unlaboured breathing and a strong regular pulse. He was perfectly stable, conscious and lucid. There was no sign of distress, in fact just the opposite; he was the calmest person in the room. The blood obviously wasn't fresh, so I reasoned that if he'd survived in this state for some time there was no need to rush anything now. But what would happen when we tried to move him? Reluctantly, I turned to the woman in the hope of getting some more information.

'When did this happen?' I asked, and then wished I hadn't.

'You tell me . . . I'm only his wife.'

'This has got to stop!' So far Mike had kept his counsel but now he moved forward and held the woman's eye. 'Can't you see how serious this is? If we ask you a question, we want a proper—'

Tony interrupted him. 'A few hours ago.'

'A few hours ago!' I was shocked. 'And since then you've just lain there in bed?'

'I didn't know what to do. I was confused. Can I have a fag?'

We both ignored him.

'Who did it to you?' Mike asked over my shoulder.

Tony remained silent.

'Tell him then, you bastard!' His wife was leaning over him now and speaking straight into his face. 'Go on, tell us all how it happened!'

I stood up and steered her away from the bed. 'Look, you're not helping things. Just tell me what's been going on here.'

She lit another cigarette and gave a resigned sigh, leaning her weight back against the wall.

'He must have got up in the night when I was asleep and gone downstairs to bother Sally. She must have done it.'

I was more confused than ever. 'Are you saying that someone stuck a knife in his neck downstairs, then he came back upstairs, got into bed and went to sleep?' She didn't reply. 'And who's Sally anyway?'

Sally, it turned out, was the woman's friend. The three of them had spent the previous evening in the pub and then come back to the house for a few more drinks. By 1 a.m. they were all a bit the worse for wear and it was decided that Sally would spend the night on the settee, and they all turned in. The inference was that some time later Sally had had an unwelcome nocturnal visitor in the form of Tony. I was beginning to get the picture, and looking more closely at the carpet I noticed spots of dried blood between the bed and the door. The trail continued out on to the landing and disappeared down the stairs. Mike was busy taking Tony's blood pressure so I decided to go down to the front room and see if I could estimate how much blood had been lost. Was the homicidal Sally still in her lair? The woman didn't know, so I asked her to come with me.

The room was in darkness but Sally's shape under a duvet on the settee was unmistakable. She didn't move when we entered but gave out a groan when the heavy curtains were drawn back and the early light filtered in.

'Sally! Sally, wake up!' The woman was shaking her shoulder while I inspected the small pool of dried blood on the carpet. It was at the end of the settee by Sally's head and that must have been where Tony was stabbed.

'Who the bloody hell's he?' Sally, her voice thick with sleep, sat up and looked at me.

'He's an ambulance man, Sal. He's come for Tony. Did you stab him?'

'Yes, I think so. Is he dead?'

She put the question so casually that she might have been enquiring how his headache was. Tony's wife, equally disdainful, put her mind at rest.

'No such luck, he's all right.'

I could hardly believe what I was listening to. Tony was lying upstairs with a knife buried in his neck, the blade of which might be nestling cosily against his carotid artery ready to rupture it at the slightest move- ment, and he was 'all right'? Would she be so relaxed if he suddenly haemorrhaged twelve pints of blood into her bed? I looked at her again and decided that she probably would be. Sally flopped back on to the sofa.

'That's OK then. Close those bloody curtains, will you!'

Tony arrived safely at the hospital lying flat on a Scoop stretcher with his neck held rigid by a cervical collar and the knife sticking out through a makeshift hole. Somehow he survived his brush with death but I would be very surprised if he came out of it any the wiser.

Piecing the story together later, it seemed he had, as suspected, crept downstairs with designs on Sally. Despite being full of drink, she was one step ahead and had made her preparations before settling down. Tony slipped into the room and leaned over her. Goodness knows what he did or said but it was enough for her to swing the knife and plunge it into his neck. He staggered away while she, satisfied that he'd learned his lesson, turned over and went back to sleep.

With his ardour dampened somewhat, Tony found himself on the horns of a dilemma. Should he wake his wife and try to explain why there was a knife embedded in his neck, or should he call an ambulance? Either way, he was going to bring down on his head the wrath of a formidable woman. He must have stood in the hall weighing up these two options with the blood trickling down when, in a flash of inspiration, he came up with a third. The obvious thing to do was to go back to bed and pretend it never happened. Maybe the knife wouldn't be there in the morning.

Chapter Eight

Mike stared moodily through the windscreen for a minute or two before breaking the silence.

'Didn't keep him out of the pub, did it?'

I looked at him. 'What didn't?'

'His ankle!'

'Oh,' I said, realizing he meant Lee, our previous patient. 'No, it didn't.'

'What time did he twist the bloody thing?'

'Eight o'clock?' I offered.

'Yeah, eight o'clock. And then what did he do?'

'Well, he—'

'I'll tell you what he bloody did.' Mike folded his arms tightly across his chest. 'He limped to the bloody pub. That's what he did. Then at chucking-out time, he limped to the takeaway. Then he limped home and ate his bloody curry. Then . . .' he paused for emphasis, 'then, at one in the bloody morning, he decides that he wants to go to hospital and has the brass neck to whistle up an ambulance to take him there! I ask you, what's the bloody world coming to?'

Having left the villain of the piece in Casualty, we were sitting in the ambulance taking a breather before contacting Control. Mike was talking more to himself than to me but I had to agree with him.

I hadn't been long in the job but I was already aware how frivolous some of the emergency calls were. That's not to say I felt able to relax. Far from it. Part of me wanted the challenge and excitement, while another part worried that I might be tested and found wanting. Would I freeze on the big occasion or, even worse, would I be reduced to a trembling liability? I had no way of knowing, and it troubled me.

Mike, on the other hand, was a grizzled veteran who had nothing to prove to anyone, least of all me. My very real fear that he might turn out to be domineering and intolerant had come to nothing; he was patience personified, content to show the way by example. If I became tongue-tied trying to deal with a difficult patient, or was left flummoxed by a tricky situation, he took over without any show of annoyance. He had an answer for everything and without him I would have been lost. I stood to attention when he spoke – jumped if he cleared his throat. He was my minder and mentor. I liked him immensely.

His tirades were another thing though. Once he launched into one there was no stopping him so on this occasion I settled back and let him get on with it, little knowing that my world was about to be turned upside down.

'And what about that bloke yesterday with his finger stuck in a pop bottle!' Mike was in full flow now. 'I mean, who in their right mind would dream of calling 999 because his finger's stuck in a bloody bottle? If ever someone deserved a good slap—'

Without warning, my door flew open, almost pitching me out of the cab. It took all my efforts to stay in my seat, and as I struggled Mike's voice boomed out over my head, 'Hey! What's your bloody game?'

'You've got to come quick!' The voice was shrill. 'It's my mate . . . I don't think he's breathing!'

A wild-eyed young man was clutching my door handle and staring beseechingly at Mike, who in turn was regarding him suspiciously. He seemed to be weighing him up, as if suspecting a prank. The moment lasted no more than a blink of the eye and when he spoke there was urgency in his tone.

'OK, son. Calm down and tell us where he is.'

'Back at the house. It's just round the corner. Please . . .' The lad could barely find the breath to say more. 'There's no time!'

With that, he took off.

'Hang on, for Christ's sake!' Mike shouted after him, but the lad was already twenty feet away and running like the wind.

Mike threw the ambulance into a jarring three-point turn and swung out of the hospital drive in time to glimpse the youth darting into a side street. My heart was beating fast. Seeing Mike transformed from the weary cynic was alarming and I almost jumped when he snapped at me, 'Come on! Get on to Control and tell them what we're doing, for heaven's sake.'

I snatched the microphone and gabbled something into it and then sat rigidly as Mike pursued the lad. He was a spent force when we caught up with him; it was all he could do to wave us towards the only illuminated house in a road of little semis. Mike accelerated past him and came to a halt among several cars abandoned at the end of the drive.

He'd barely pulled on the handbrake before a woman broke away from a group on the doorstep and came running down the path towards us. At first I couldn't make out what she was shouting but, as she got closer, her words took shape.

'He's dead! He's dead!'

Instinctively I looked to Mike, only to find that he was already out of the ambulance and reaching behind the driver's seat for his emergency case. When he spoke there was an edge to his voice I hadn't heard before.

'Bring the oxygen.'

My heart thumped. Right, oxygen. I fumbled stupidly with the fastenings before getting the case clear and then ran to the house. Mike had disappeared inside and someone shouted, 'Upstairs! Quick, upstairs!'

I heard the panic in the voice and, disconcertingly, I felt some of it move into me.

A small child was peering down from a sea of legs on the landing as I reached the foot of the stairs. Her eyes held mine for a moment, then widened in alarm as an arm swooped down and whisked her away. A moment later I was on the landing being pulled towards a room on my left by a man old enough to be my father. He was telling me that his son wasn't breathing and to hurry. I had to stay calm but my legs were trembling when I met Mike at the bedroom door. He was steering a woman from the room; she couldn't have been more than twenty-five and her tear-stained face almost brushed mine as she passed. A man behind me took hold of her and began talking rapidly into her ear, trying to reassure her.

'The ambulance is here, it's going to be OK . . . It's going to be OK . . . The ambulance is here now.'

Mike had turned back into the bedroom and was leaning over the body of a young man on the bed. There was only time for me to glimpse fixed eyes staring from a grey face before a sudden thunder of feet on the stairs made me swing round. A man not much older than me exploded into the room. Fear was etched on his face.

'Vic! Vic!'

He fell to his knees by the bed. Mike turned and looked at me in exasperation and said something. I think he was telling me to get the man out, but when

I reached out and touched his shoulder, saying that we needed space to work, the man violently jerked my hand away.

'He's my brother! Do something for him!'

I couldn't find any words. I was still searching for them when the young woman rushed back in. She barged against Mike in an effort to reach the bed. He shrugged her off and, raising his voice, demanded that the room be cleared. Turning to me again, he rasped out that I should get everyone to move away. But I had no authority; they wouldn't listen to me. I was floundering when an older voice rose above the others.

'Let them do their job!' He kept repeating the words. 'Let them do their job, let them do their job.' It was his sheer persistence that made the man and woman stand back and then leave the room.

Now I could get to Mike's side, I started scrabbling at the oxygen bag. Things fell from it as I tried to switch on the cylinder. Despite my shaking hands, I managed to turn the key. I looked at Mike for instructions but he was leaning back from the body, shaking his head.

'You can forget the oxygen,' he said quietly.

Forget it? 'But Mike, surely we must try . . . We must do something.'

'He's had it. He's dead. There's nothing we can do.'

Car doors were slamming outside, followed by more raised voices and the clatter of a woman's shoes on the path.

'We must do something,' I repeated.

Mike turned on me and hissed, 'For God's sake! We're going to have enough trouble with the family, I don't need you adding to it. Look!' Lifting the sheet, he grabbed the man's wrist and pulled it towards him. There was slight but obvious resistance at the elbow. 'Rigor mortis! Can you see it? He's starting to stiffen. He's been dead for hours!'

Mike pulled the sheet back into place and got to his feet.

'I'm going to tell the family that we're too late to do anything for him. You can gather up our stuff.' With that, he went back out on to the landing.

A few moments later Mike extinguished any flicker of hope our arrival had raised. Above the collective groan of despair that swept through the house, a woman wailed like a wounded animal.

'No! No! No! Not my son!'

I caught only a fleeting image of her as she burst into the bedroom and collapsed on to the young man. I was appalled and frightened by her screams. I could smell her perfume as she looked up at me.

'Do something for him, he needs you!' she shouted. 'Oh God in heaven, what's happening? Why are you just standing there?'

For a moment I thought she was going to attack me and I backed away, but she turned back to her son and screamed again, 'No, No, No!'

All I could do was watch as her husband took

her by the shoulders and guided her out of the room.

I followed them out, to find that the little girl had reappeared by one of the bedroom doors. Her lips were trembling and she stared at me as if I were a monster. I couldn't look at her. Her father – it had to be her father – was dead and there was nothing I could do. I turned away to see Mike standing almost nose-to-nose with the hysterical mother. She had her back against the wall and he had his arms either side of her, forming a cage that she couldn't escape from. He wasn't touching her but she couldn't move and, as Mike spoke, her moans turned to whimpers. I couldn't hear what he was saying but his words seemed to penetrate; she became quieter, and then sobbed silently.

Claustrophobic and with no other thought but escape, I headed for the stairs, keeping my eyes fixed on the carpet as I squeezed past people. Some of them spoke to me but I didn't answer. Once outside I took a deep breath of cold air. What was I doing here in the midst of all this grief? I felt anger and resentment. This wasn't the deal; this wasn't why I had joined the ambulance service. I was supposed to be saving people, not declaring them dead. And the hysteria – I'd never experienced anything like it before. It was intimidating but, worse than that, it was infectious. I hadn't been prepared for it, how could I have been? I also cursed my own inadequacy. Mike was still in the house with the relatives while I was hiding in the front garden. It must have been ten minutes before I found the courage to go back inside.

Mike was coming down the stairs looking tired and drawn.

'Oh, there you are,' he said without irony. 'Look, I'm going to get on the radio and ask for a doctor to come out and certify the lad.' Then he added, 'Have you brought our stuff down from the bedroom?'

I'd forgotten all about it.

'No, not yet. I was just going to get it,' I lied.

'OK. Go and fetch it, then I think it might be an idea to keep out of the way and wait in the ambulance.'

The atmosphere in the house had changed. A hush had descended; most people were in groups, talking in lowered voices, while a few sat alone. Through the open kitchen door I could see a woman trying to fill a kettle, her hand shaking so much that most of the water found its way into the sink. Then, once again, I was on the landing and found myself looking around for the little girl, but she wasn't there. In the bedroom the dead man's mother and a younger woman were sitting by the body. Neither looked up as I collected our bags.

By the front door I was stopped by a middle-aged man wearing an anorak thrown over a pair of pyjamas.

'Thanks for all you've done.' If there had been a hint of sarcasm in his voice I would probably have bolted. As it was, I just stared at him as he continued. 'Say thanks to your mate for me as well. He deserves it.'

The very idea of being thanked when we had done nothing was bizarre. I started to babble.

'Look, there's nothing to thank us for. We didn't do anything . . . I wish we could have but—'

He held up a hand. 'Didn't do anything? Your mate did a lot. I'm just a neighbour but even I knew there was no bringing Vic back. I don't know how we would have coped with the family if your mate hadn't been there. Whatever he said to Vic's mother worked. He even went round the rest of the family and spoke to them one by one. He's a good man, just tell him that from me.'

Back in the cab I let out a long, slow breath.

'They appreciated you, Mike. I was told to say thanks to you.'

He gave me an incredulous look. 'What on earth for?'

'The way you looked after the mother and relatives. I couldn't have done it. I didn't know what to do or say, I just went blank. I'm sorry I was useless.'

'There was nothing either of us could do. It was all over long before we got there.'

'Yes, I know. I mean I was no help to you . . . It just kind of overwhelmed me.'

'Listen!' He turned in his seat and faced me. 'You've only been in the job five minutes, I wouldn't have expected anything else from you. It wasn't made any easier with so many of the family turning up.'

'Yes, but—'

'There's no room for any bloody "buts". These things happen. Learn from it and put it behind you.' His tone softened a little. 'Take it from me, if you brood on it you'll just go round in circles. I should know, I've gone round in plenty of circles in my time.'

'You say he was only twenty-four?'

'Yes.'

'That's just a year older than me,' I said.

Mike looked back out through the windscreen and said nothing.

'Do you know what happened . . . why he died?' I couldn't leave it alone.

A hint of irritation returned to Mike's voice. 'I'm not a bloody pathologist. All I know is that he was asthmatic, so the chances are that's what it was. It could have been anything though.'

'What I don't understand,' I said, 'is how he could have been dead so long before anyone found him? I mean, where was his wife?'

Mike sighed. 'The story I got was that he'd gone to bed at about half seven, saying he didn't feel too good. His wife put it down to a touch of the flu and thought no more of it. She didn't go upstairs until the late film finished on telly some time after two, when she found him on the bed with the sheets on the floor. She must have known that he was dead and ran next door, where one of the lad's friends lives. He came round, took one look, shot out the house and legged it round to the hospital. It didn't cross the daft bugger's mind to pick up the phone.'

When I got home Marie was bustling around getting ready to leave for work. She was running late and didn't ask her customary question, 'How did your night go?' I was grateful, and went to bed still wrestling with the concept of a young life ending with no more ceremony than the snuffing out of a candle. I knew there was little point in looking for rhyme or reason and, as Mike said, these things happen. If I was going to survive in this job I would just have to get used to it.

Chapter Nine

As the weeks passed it became clear that Henrietta Street was anything but the penal colony I'd been led to expect. In fact, it proved to be quite the opposite. I saw it as a wonderful, vibrant depot staffed by the best bunch of people I'd ever met. Most were a good bit older than me and had served in the forces before finding their way into the ambulance service. Some had fought in the Second World War and then in Korea. Mike carried a scar received on D-Day when a bullet hit him in the hand and exited further up on his forearm, leaving him with a withered thumb. Joe Haynes had been in a bomb disposal team, sent into Bergen-Belsen concentration camp to check for booby traps before anyone else was allowed to enter. Others had seen active service in Palestine, Kenya, Malaya, Borneo and all corners of the empire.

This predominance of ex-servicemen gave the place a sense of discipline, but what struck me most forcibly was the 'can do' mentality everyone seemed imbued with. Self-sufficiency was a byword. Woe betide anyone who called for assistance out on the road unless it was indisputably essential. I dare say it would be written off as macho posturing these days, but it wasn't that; it had more to do with personal pride and the fear of 'not measuring up'. Loyalty among the staff was fierce. Problems were sorted out on the shift and the only time the manager found someone knocking on his door was when he'd messed up the leave rota. Even then you had to think carefully before tangling with him. He'd been a chief petty officer in the navy and it was child's play for him to reduce someone like me to a quivering wreck. But he was loyal to us; it would have been a brave person who criticized his depot within his hearing. Perhaps it was this 'band of brothers' mentality, coupled with the tough inner-city environment in which we worked, that led outsiders to view the Street with apprehension and even suspicion.

I moved through this strange new world in a constant state of wonder. Everyone else had seen and done so much more than me. Late night conversations often ranged over events and places beyond my ken, leaving me only able to contribute a laugh or a groan when required. I mean, what could I add when the topic was how best to defend yourself against vagabonds in the back streets of Nairobi? What could I do but listen when a couple of them started exchanging reminiscences of storming hills in Korea? As a newcomer, I was even left out in the cold when it came to discussing ambulance work.

This was brought home to me one evening when Mike and I came back on station to the sound of laughter coming from the messroom. Larry was on his feet talking and broke off as we entered.

'Oh, hi Mike, I was just telling the others about this job we've just done.'

Mike slumped into his usual seat. 'Carry on, don't mind me.'

'Well, as I was saying, we called at this house and a bloke of about sixty opens the door holding a cloth soaked in blood and snot to his mouth. It looked like he'd been punched, but he mumbled something about his dog having done it. Then he goes and sticks a handful of broken teeth and fillings under my nose. Bloody disgusting it was, almost made me throw up.' Larry grimaced at the memory. 'Anyway, you know how me and dogs don't get on. I suddenly got worried and asked him where it was, only for the silly sod to open the living-room door and say, "in here". Before I knew what was happening, out leaps the biggest Staffordshire bull terrier you've ever seen.' Larry held his arms out expansively to illustrate the point. 'Its chest was the size of a fridge freezer and its head was bigger than a medicine ball. I swear I could have climbed on its back and ridden it round the room. I thought my number was up but it turned out to be as daft as a brush. It just barged about with its tongue hanging out and its tail going like a windmill.'

'That's a shame,' Steve said. 'This might have been worth listening to if it had gone for you.'

'If it had gone for me I wouldn't be here to tell the story. You'd be bringing me flowers in intensive care.'

'OK, get on with it.' Steve was getting impatient. 'How does a dog manage to knock someone's teeth out?'

Larry smiled. 'This is where it gets really stupid. Ben, that's the bloke, came back from the pub after a few pints and thought it would be a good idea to play a game with Billy, that's the dog—'

'Ben and Billy?' Steve interrupted. 'Bill and Ben? You've got to be joking.'

Larry faltered; he obviously hadn't twigged any connection to the Flowerpot Men of *Watch with Mother* fame.

'So which one was the dog? Was it Bill or was it Ben?' Steve laughed at his own joke.

'Just shut up, will you!' Larry waited for silence. 'So, Ben fetches Billy's rubber play ring but then, instead of holding it in his hand and having a game of tug, he gets down on all fours and makes like a dog.'

'You're not going to tell us he put the bloody ring in his mouth?' Mike said.

'That's exactly what he did.' Larry grinned. 'And not only that, once he's got it clamped between his teeth he starts making growling sounds. Just shows how a couple of beers can cloud your judgement. I mean, at sixty his teeth couldn't have been in the best nick anyway. Billy wouldn't hurt a fly but at the end of the day a dog's a dog, isn't it? So,' Larry continued, 'Billy grips hold of his side of the ring and straight away pulls Ben off balance. For the life of me I don't know why Ben didn't see the light there and then. But, needless to say, he didn't. To avoid being dragged across the room, he hung on even harder – just as Billy gave the ring a shake that would have broken a small animal's neck. Before the silly sod knew what was happening, his teeth had disintegrated and exploded out of his mouth like a hailstorm.'

Larry shook his head. 'I tell you, I'm glad I wasn't there to see it happen. When I shone my pen torch in his mouth it looked like a hand grenade had gone off in there. All I could see through the blood was stumps and holes. Some of his teeth were pulled out whole while others, top and bottom, were snapped off at the gum. He'll be finding them round the room for days.' This brought snorts of distaste from the others that quickly turned to hoots of derision when Larry added piously, 'It just goes to show the perils of drink.' It seemed Larry was notorious for spending a fair bit of his leisure time in the pub.

As always, one story inspires another, and over the next half-hour everyone chipped in with at least one dog story of their own. Everyone but me, that is. When the conversation eventually began to lag I saw my chance to tell the tale of the man with the knife buried in his neck. It didn't have anything to do with dogs but it struck me as the kind of event that might generate a bit of interest. It took all of two seconds for me to realize I'd made a bad mistake.

Gerald had warned me in training to keep my head down and my mouth shut and I quickly discovered it was probably the best piece of advice he'd given me. It was just too presumptuous for someone only a few weeks into the job to try and impress a group of people with one hundred and twenty years' experience between them. If I'd just saved the Pope's life no one would have listened. Steve picked up a newspaper and, while a couple of the others exchanged weary looks, Larry asked if anyone wanted a cup of tea. I began to lose the thread, my neck went hot and if the ground had swallowed me up I would have been eternally grateful. Mike, as usual, came to my rescue. He saw the hole I was digging for myself and subtly took over the story. He immediately gained everyone's full attention and I slunk off into the kitchen to make the pot of tea Larry had suggested.

Mike and I did one more job before the end of the shift, and Larry's warning of the 'perils of drink' popped into my head as soon as we met the patient. We'd been called to help a woman who'd fallen in her garden and couldn't get back on her feet. It was quite a house. Three white marble steps flanked by wrought-iron railings led up to the front door, and despite the windswept autumn evening we couldn't help but stop a moment to look around in admiration. From the gravel drive that swept past immaculate lawns and well-established trees, to the double-fronted Edwardian house, everything oozed solid, middle-class respectability. Mike lifted the brass knocker and let it fall back with a heavy *thunk*. A few seconds later the door opened halfway and the impish face of a girl of about ten peeped round.

'Hi-ya. You were quick, come in.'

After closing the door she turned to us with what might have been an apologetic look.

'I'm sorry to have called you. Mummy's a lot better now. She's come in from the garden and just wants to go to bed.'

Mike looked down at her and smiled. 'That's OK. My name's Mike, by the way. What's yours?'

'Fiona,' she replied brightly.

'OK, Fiona. Now that we're here anyway, do you think we could have a quick word with your mum?'

'Yes of course. She's awfully tired, but I know she won't mind.'

We followed as she skipped down the oak-panelled hall and through to the kitchen.

We found her mother sitting on the floor propped up against the washing machine. Her legs were drawn up tightly against her body and her chin rested on a muddy knee protruding through a large tear in her dress. She opened her eyes and looked up as we came in.

'Who are they, Fiona?'

'It's the ambulance men, Mummy. I called them

when you fell over in the garden. Don't you remember?'

'Anbuli . . . Ambilansh?' She gave up and a slow, lazy smile spread across her face, only to fade as her eyelids drooped shut again. I'd been alarmed by the state of her at first, but that smile told its own story: it was the unmistakable smile of someone who was completely sozzled. Under normal circumstances she would have been a handsome woman. She was slim with elegant features and, it has to be said, fitted very nicely into a clinging black gown. At her throat was a gold necklace, which was complemented by matching bracelets and earrings. I guessed her to be about forty.

Mike knelt down at her side and spoke firmly to gain her attention. 'Hello, I'm Mike. What's your name?'

She opened her eyes and squinted at him, then slowly raised a forefinger and waggled it in his general direction.

'My name? Now that . . . would be telling . . . wouldn't it.'

'Why are you sitting on the floor?' Mike asked, taking her pulse.

She seemed to be trying to focus on him.

'Why not? Itch a free world. Ishntit?'

'Oh Mummy, you are being so rude!' Fiona folded her arms across her chest disapprovingly and looked at Mike. 'Her name's Victoria.'

'Come on then, Victoria,' Mike said. 'Let's get you off the floor.'

Working together, we helped her to her feet and supported her the two or three steps to a kitchen chair. Once sitting, she took a deep breath and tried to regain some dignity by carefully and deliberately crossing her legs and unsuccessfully attempting to brush a wayward lock of hair from her eyes.

'How are you feeling now?' Mike asked.

'Oh . . . you know . . . you know . . .' Her voice tailed off as she fiddled with her hair again.

'Come on, Victoria, at least try and speak to me.'

She took another deep breath, and slurred, 'Mo K, thanks. Why all the fush? Why's everyone fushing so?'

Her breath put me in mind of a public bar just before closing time.

Mike turned to Fiona. 'Shall we get your mum upstairs to bed?'

She gave it a moment's thought and said, 'Yes, I think that's a good idea. She's very tired.'

Her mother had now taken a keen interest in the tear in her dress and was pulling the edges together, seemingly in the hope they might rejoin. Mike and I took an elbow each and, with Fiona leading the way, helped her upstairs to the bedroom. She was asleep before the covers were pulled over her.

Back downstairs, Fiona took us through to the lounge. 'Coffee?'

We accepted, partly as it gave us time to decide what to do next. Leaving a ten-year-old girl in charge of an inebriated adult probably broke some law or other.

When she came back with the drinks Mike tackled her.

'Where's your dad then?'

'Daddy? Oh, he's at the golf club. There are always lots of people he has to see. He won't be long, he's usually back by nine.'

As it was nearly nine o'clock, we decided to wait in the hope he'd be home on time. Fiona went off to check on her mother, leaving us to admire the expensively furnished but cosy room. It was a far cry from most of the houses we found ourselves in and I stood up to admire what looked to be an original David Shepherd lion painting hanging above the large marble fireplace. I was leaning forward to get a closer look when a key sounded in the front door.

The sound of Fiona greeting her father in the entrance hall filtered through and a moment later she led him into the lounge without warning him we were there. He was a rotund little man in grey slacks and a navy blue blazer that sported a large club badge on the breast pocket. He hesitated slightly on seeing us, but quickly regained his composure.

'Hello, chaps, this is a bit of a surprise. I saw an ambulance outside but I assumed it was for old Mrs Kent next door.' He looked at Fiona. 'What's been happening? Is it Mummy again, sugar pie?'

'Yes, she's had a bit of a funny turn,' Fiona said.

'Really. What was it this time?'

'She went into the garden for some fresh air and fell

over. She's fine now, I just checked on her. She's tucked up in bed like a little lamb.'

Her father took in the information with little show of surprise or disquiet.

'Good girl, that's the ticket.' Then, looking at us, he lowered his voice. 'She has these turns every now and then, you know . . . Can't be helped.'

'Daddy, just look at your tie, it's all over the place!' Fiona reached up and began readjusting it. 'I hope you weren't sitting in the club looking like this.'

'Really, sweetie, there's no need to bother . . .'

'And I made you a sandwich for when you got back. It's in the fridge.'

'Thank you, sweetie, you're an angel.'

While his tie was being straightened he returned his attention to us.

'Sit down, chaps, sit down. I see Fiona's sorted you out with a coffee.'

With his tie rearranged to Fiona's satisfaction, he lowered himself into a large leather armchair while she perched on the armrest.

'Well then . . . here we are.' He had one of those rich, plummy voices. 'I'm sorry you've been dragged out for nothing. Has it been a busy night?'

Within a couple of minutes we felt like old family friends who'd called in unexpectedly.

When Mike managed to steer the conversation back to the woman slumbering upstairs her husband seemed curiously unconcerned.

'She'll be fine. She takes on far too much these days. I'm sure it's just a case of overtiredness, don't you agree?'

Mike, aware Fiona was glued to every word, seemed unsure of what to say. 'Well, erm . . .'

Fiona had her own thoughts on the subject. 'If you ask me, Daddy, I think she's pissed again.'

Her father looked at her in horror. 'Fiona! Really! Where on earth did you learn to talk like that?'

'That's what you always say when she's like this, Daddy. Pissed again, you say.'

'Fiona! Enough!' His tone was abrupt but quickly mellowed. 'Darling, please, that's enough. Anyway, she can't have been drinking. We don't keep any of the hard stuff in the house any more.' He looked over at us. 'Best not to tempt fate, if you know what I mean.'

Fiona was indignant. 'Yes we do, Daddy! Mummy always has something to drink. She keeps it in the organ.'

'In the organ, darling? Don't be silly. I mean, how could she? No, that's simply not on.'

'She does, Daddy! I'll show you.' With that she jumped from the arm of the chair and headed for the door.

Her father stood up and, glancing across at us, gave an exaggerated sigh as he followed her out. Mike and I exchanged a look and decided to tag along. We crossed the hall and entered another reception room, where I was immediately stopped in my tracks. Standing alone in the otherwise empty room was a full-size church organ, the golden glow of its ancient polished oak burning hot against the pale grey carpet and walls. It was far larger than the door aperture and must have been dismantled and then reassembled in the room. Why was it there? What possible function could it perform? There were no pipes or any other means for it to make a significant sound. I looked questioningly at Mike as if he might have the answer. His face was impassive as he spoke from the corner of his mouth.

'Don't even ask.'

While I pondered the sheer incongruity of what I was looking at, Fiona ran over and squatted down among the foot pedals. Obviously enjoying the drama of the moment, she removed a panel from the back board and reached inside to pull out a bottle of vodka, which she held triumphantly above her head.

'Here it is, Daddy.'

We walked over and peered into the aperture; it was an Aladdin's cave. Bottles of spirits, wine, packets of peanuts and biscuits, a bottle opener and drinking glasses were stashed away in the depths. We all looked at each other. Fiona, still holding the vodka, was beaming. Her father obviously knew nothing of the illicit cache and was momentarily lost for words.

'What in the name of . . . ?' His voice trailed off, then found itself again. 'Well, well, well, the cunning . . .' He looked back in at the bottles. With a slow grin spreading across his face, he shook his head and muttered, 'Very clever! Good for you, old thing, good for you.' Then, turning to us, 'Fancy a proper drink, chaps? It'll be on the house.'

Chapter Ten

It must have been around three in the morning when Larry slipped purposefully into the messroom, crossed to his seat in two bounds and snatched up a newspaper. A few suspicious heads turned in his direction but before anyone could ask what he'd been up to Howard appeared in the doorway, tight-lipped and red in the face. He held a mound of snooker balls in each hand.

'Not funny!'

As he spoke, the black ball slipped from his grasp, bounced on the floor and, as if by instinct, rolled into a corner of the room.

'What's not funny, H?' Mike asked in genuine bemusement.

'Stupid pranks, Mike . . . stupid pranks that could get someone hurt!' He looked at each of us in turn. 'I don't know which one of you it was, but I tell you this . . . if it ever happens again I'll find the pea-brained bastard and personally stuff these balls down his throat. Am I making myself clear?'

No one said anything. After another prolonged stare, H threw the remaining snooker balls on to the table and delivered a parting shot before stomping out of the room.

'Make no mistake . . . I'll stuff them down his throat!'

We sat in silence as his footsteps faded down the corridor, then Steve gave a low whistle.

'Bloody hell, I've never seen H lose his temper before. What on earth did you do to him, Larry?'

'Me?'

'Yes, you!'

Larry shifted uncomfortably. 'It was only the old snooker-ball thing in the bog. I don't know why he's got so worked up about it.'

Using the toilet late at night was a perilous business. The only chance of being left in peace was to lay a false trail, such as announcing you were off to hoover your car or restock the ambulance. If the real reason for your disappearance was discovered, you were in trouble. While the intended victim sat in the stall, alert as a nervous gazelle, the prankster would silently open the outer door and, when he felt confident that he hadn't been detected, would raise the metal waste-paper bin and crash it down on the tiled floor with all the strength at his command. The hope was that the reverberating crash would induce a heart attack in the victim. A refinement on the same theme was to take in an armful of snooker balls and hurl them across the floor. This created a sudden hailstorm of noise with the gratifying bonus of inflicting a little pain as the balls bounced round the ankles and shins of the hapless victim.

I learned all this later the hard way, but for now I was perplexed. Steve understood all too well but was still unconvinced by Larry's explanation.

'He wouldn't have got so mad if that's all you did.'

'His trouble is that he can't take a joke any more,' Larry responded. 'Did you hear me complain when he tied a kipper to the engine of my ambulance? It stank for days! And it's not as if it wasn't premeditated either. You don't just come across a kipper by accident and then wonder . . . hmm, what shall I do with this.'

'So,' Steve said, 'it wasn't premeditated when you sprinkled curry powder into the air vents of his motor the week before? Anyway, you're getting off the subject. How have you managed to upset H so badly?'

Larry looked pained and lit a cigarette. 'Well, maybe I shouldn't have, but I thought it would be a new twist if, instead of just rolling the balls across the floor, I threw them over the top of the cubicle.'

Steve's eyes widened. 'What? You dropped a load of snooker balls five feet on to his head while he was sitting on the toilet? You can't be serious!'

'I suppose it was a bit stupid. It was funny though – you should have heard him yelp.'

'Funny! You could have killed him! If you'd done it

to anyone else but H, you'd be in the back of your own ambulance on the way to hospital by now.'

Mike looked over his glasses and wrapped up the conversation.

'Just a word of warning, Larry. If you try anything like that again it'll be me who's stuffing you full of snooker balls, and it won't be by way of your mouth.'

I'd maintained my new-found code of silence more in amazement than by design. Here we were, a supposedly intelligent, responsible group of adults, and none of us safe from a stream of practical jokes, the like of which wouldn't have tested the ingenuity of your average schoolboy. These 'jokes' were part and parcel of working at the Street and mostly taken in good heart. If anything, they were seen by the victim as the perfect excuse to plan what sometimes turned out to be quite elaborate revenge. Howard's reaction though, even if perfectly understandable, took everyone by surprise. H, or to give him his proper name, Howard Hallam, was the nicest, calmest, most even-tempered person you could wish to meet and, until that moment, I don't think anyone thought it possible he could lose his temper.

Slightly chubby with a mop of permanently ruffled blond hair, H was one of those people you couldn't help but like. He simply radiated bonhomie wherever he went. It took only a casual glance in his direction to induce a smile that lit his face up like a pinball machine; even something trivial, like making him a cup of tea, would earn such gratitude you were left feeling quite dazed. It's not easy to remain universally popular in a world of strong-minded, not to say opinionated people, but H pulled it off consummately. And even the patients loved him. How could they fail to when he made them feel so special? No matter how trivial their problem might be, he could be relied on to give it his undivided attention. In fact, he went further than that; he actively encouraged them to pour out their smallest medical woes and then sat back in open-mouthed fascination while they got on with it. Hearing that old Mrs Brown's bunion, contracted in 1952, was still giving her gyp all these years later was enough to induce frowns of genuine concern and sympathy. Money couldn't buy such an appreciative audience, and the patients knew it.

I'd been working with him for the past week and had been made to feel welcome from the start. Despite being at least ten years older, and with nine years' experience under his belt, he'd gone to such lengths to be friendly that I began to imagine he felt privileged having me as a partner. It was a nonsensical notion, but that's how Howard made everybody feel. What struck me most forcibly, though, was his total commitment to the job, and the obvious pleasure he took in passing on his knowledge. This was lucky for me as my conversation at the time consisted solely of nervous openers like 'What would you do if . . . ?' or 'How would you treat such-and-such?' He would patiently weigh each naive question as if it were startlingly original and then launch into detailed answers. But, as everyone constantly reminded me, the only true way to learn was through experience.

So far I'd been fortunate in finding myself plunged into unusual situations, and the week I spent with Howard didn't buck the trend. A few nights earlier we'd been called to a man who'd fallen through an open hatch on his canal boat. There are miles of canals criss-crossing Birmingham, though you would scarcely notice unless you went looking for them. The city grew up round them, and then engulfed them; but they're still there, albeit mostly hidden from sight. A few mooring points are scattered round the system and in the centre there's a decent-sized wharf where a few hardy types live on permanently moored boats. That's where we were headed, and a pretty dingy, slimy place it was back then.

A man was waiting by the short gangplank to one of the longboats. He looked cold, despite being buried inside an oversize sheepskin coat.

'He's down there.' He pointed towards a small black hole in the deck towards the bow. 'We'd just got back from the pub and he was showing me round the boat when he suddenly vanished. I thought he'd gone over the side until I heard him shouting.'

We picked our way down the deck and H peered into the darkness of the hatch.

'Are you OK down there?'

'No, I'm fucking not! It's my leg . . . I think it's bust.'

'OK. Just sit tight and we'll get some light on the situation.'

'I haven't got much choice, have I . . . and don't strike any matches, for God's sake. There's diesel slopping about down here.'

The few lights along the wharf barely had the energy to reflect off the murky water and, thanks to our station manager, I didn't expect much more of our torches. One of his more baffling quirks, and he had no shortage of them, was an almost pathological dread of parting with anything from the station stores. In particular, he guarded the torch batteries as if they were made of weapons-grade plutonium. This was all very well for balancing his budget, but it meant that when I directed my torch into the hold the only real effect it had was to turn the darkness vaguely orange.

'Blimey, when did you last change the batteries?' H asked.

'I tried to get some new ones the other day, but the boss told me they didn't grow on trees and to clear off.'

'Hmm, that sounds like him. He can be like that with new people.' H pulled out his own torch and switched it on. 'You should stand your ground though. You can look a right pillock if the batteries fa—' The beam he was casting had suddenly faded and flickered out. 'Bloody hell!' He banged the torch against the deck in the vain hope of reviving it. 'Oh well, we'll just have to make do with yours. Keep it on while I climb down and check this character over.'

The hatch wasn't much more than two feet square, so H had some difficulty in squeezing his bulk through. Among the clutter below I could make out old jerrycans, coils of rope and, taking up much of the space, what I guessed to be an iron winding mechanism. Beside this lay our patient, who looked to be in his late twenties and dressed in a similar fashion to his friend. I dropped the torch down to H and waited while he checked for injuries. I couldn't hear much of the mumbled conversation until the quiet of the night was rudely shattered.

'*Whaaaargh!*'

'Is that where the pain is?' Howard's voice was measured, leaving me unsure if he was being serious, ironic, or just taking a little revenge for being sworn at earlier.

'You bloody bet it is . . . Jesus!'

Howard straightened up, bringing his head level with the hatch.

'He's displaced his kneecap. There doesn't seem to be much else wrong with him, but I can't be sure. I'm afraid we'll have to keep him flat in case he's buggered his back in the fall.'

'Keep him flat? How are we going to get him out of there if he can't bend? We need another crew to help, don't we?'

'Let's not jump the gun. If you'll go and fetch the

Neil Robinson we'll see if we can work something out.' With that he disappeared back down into the orange glow.

The Neil Robinson is a rescue stretcher made from a stout canvas sheet held rigid along its length by a series of wooden slats stitched into the material. When the patient's been manoeuvred on to it, it's then moulded to his body shape before being secured by leather straps. Only the face is left visible, and he can't move a muscle. Not the kind of device to warm the heart of a claustrophobic, but handy for rescue work.

The glow coming from the hold had noticeably waned when I got back to the boat. H popped his head out and took one end of the stretcher to pull it inside. I followed it in, trying my best to ignore the sickly sweet smell of oil and diesel.

H kicked various obstacles in his path into the shadows and managed to wedge the Neil Robinson in beside the patient. Everything seemed to be covered in grease, and every movement brought us into contact with something hard. The dwindling light didn't help much either, but H had an idea as we struggled to get the man immobilized.

'You must have a torch in the boat. Can your mate go and fetch it before ours pegs out?'

There was a pause. 'I don't have the cabin keys on me.'

'You don't have the keys? Well, where are they? Has your mate got them?'

Another pause. 'I don't think so.'

'That's a bit strange, isn't it?' Howard continued talking as we manhandled the stretcher over the iron winder and to a position near the hatch. 'How were you going to get in?'

'Well . . .'

My torch finally gave up the ghost and Howard sighed. 'That's a nuisance.'

Our eyes had become pretty well accustomed to the poor conditions and the light filtering down from the wharf made it possible to pick out shapes in the darkness. Even so, I was starting to feel uncomfortable and wondered what H was going to do now.

'Maybe it's time to call for another ambulance?' I said in his general direction. 'I mean, even if we could see what we were doing, how are we supposed to get him up on deck?'

'That shouldn't be a problem—' He swore as he slipped on the goo underfoot. 'To start with, we have to get him more or less upright and prop him against the bulkhead. From there it'll be a piece of cake.'

The patient was pretty scrawny but even so it was hard work in the confined space, and by the time we had him in position I was gasping for breath.

'Right, that was easy enough,' H said. 'The idea now is for two of us to push from below while the other pulls from above. You get out on deck and send his mate down.'

He didn't need to ask twice.

It hadn't crossed my mind to draft in his mate to help and by the affronted look he gave me it hadn't crossed his either. He took off his coat and, grumbling all the way, climbed down into the boat as if he were being sent into the black hole of Calcutta. I could hear H giving instructions and then, amid grunts and groans, one end of the stretcher slowly inched into view. I grabbed the rope handles and heaved while they pushed. Bit by bit the patient came up into the land of the living and when his feet were clear I was able to lay him flat on the deck. He stared at the stars and let out a long sigh.

'Thank Christ for that. I was sure you were going to drop me.'

I'd been expecting a 'thank you', and had already prepared a response along the lines of 'Don't mention it, mate, that's what we're here for.' Instead, I contented myself by looking down at my diesel-soaked trousers and grease-smeared shirt, wondering what Marie was going to say when she saw them.

Howard's uniform was in a similar state but he seemed more interested in speaking to the patient than in his own appearance.

'This isn't your boat, is it?'

The man flicked his eyes towards him. 'What do you mean? Of course it's my boat!'

'Why haven't you got the keys for it then?'

'What is this? My leg's killing me and you're more interested in the boat?'

Howard wasn't to be put off. 'If it is your boat, then tell me its name.'

'Its name?'

'Yes, its name. All boats have names.'

The man returned his gaze to the stars and said nothing.

'You didn't even fall down the hatch, did you? You'd have more injuries if you'd dropped into that lot. I reckon you were down there looking for something to nick and tripped in the dark.'

The man kept his silence.

'What I can't understand,' H continued, 'is why you came up with a cock-and-bull story about falling in. All the trouble we went to! If I'd known from the start it was just your knee, you'd have been out in minutes. I should call the police.'

The patient looked back at H. 'Well done, Sherlock. It's a fair cop,' he said sarcastically. 'The fall was my mate's idea; he thought it would explain why I was down there. And if you want to call the police, feel free . . . They couldn't even do me for trespass.'

H rubbed the bridge of his nose, leaving a greasy smudge between his eyes, and scanned the wharf.

'Some mate. He's disappeared faster than a rat up a drainpipe.' He looked at me and shook his head. 'Come on then, Les, let's get him to hospital.'

As we sat in the ambulance later, H said, 'That's been a good lesson for you. Never take anything at face value. I don't know if I'm getting old or what, but it wasn't till we were pushing him through the hatch that the penny dropped. I suppose there was one saving grace though.'

'Oh, what's that?' I asked.

'We didn't call out another crew. Can you imagine what Mike and Larry would have made of it when they found it was only a burglar with a dislocated knee? We'd never have heard the end of it.'

Later that week H and I found ourselves embroiled in another case which proved more complex than a first glance suggested. The incident was given over the radio as a road traffic accident involving only one car. It was about seven in the evening but already dark. The conditions were good and there was no obvious reason why the car should have left the road. But there it was, straddling the pavement with its back wheels in the gutter and its bonnet jammed up against a garden wall. Other than a broken headlight and bent bumper and grille, there seemed to be little wrong with it. Whoever had been driving had disappeared, leaving the driver's door hanging open in a way that suggested the car had been hastily abandoned after the crash. Stolen cars are involved in a lot of accidents; sometimes as a result of reckless driving, but often it boils down to deliberate vandalism.

A police car was parked near by and the officer was inspecting the damage by torchlight. Howard, reluctant to leave the warmth of the cab for no good reason, wound down his window and shouted over, 'Done a runner, have they?'

The officer switched off his torch and looked up.

'I've just got here myself, but one of the kids from the house says there's an injured woman inside.' He gestured over the wall towards the large terraced house set back some seven or eight feet from the pavement. 'I haven't spoken to her yet. If you want to go and check her over I'll join you when I've radioed this through.' He looked back at the car with a shake of the head. 'Women drivers! How on earth did she manage this?'

Considering the light damage to the car, and that the woman had felt up to walking to the house, I grabbed my first aid bag and headed down the path, confident this would be a case I could manage without Howard feeling it necessary to look over my shoulder.

A girl of about eight met us in the hallway. She was trembling and spoke in a small voice as she gestured towards the living room.

'The lady's in there.'

'Thanks.' I made a move towards the door.

'She's bleeding, will you look after her?' The child was on the point of tears and I took a moment to reassure her.

'Of course we'll look after her. She'll soon be as right as rain.' The girl didn't look convinced. 'Don't worry,' I said, and carried on into the living room, 'we fix people's cuts all the time.'

Standing by the fireplace opposite the door was a

woman with her arm round an even younger child. She was deathly pale and, without raising her eyes in my direction, nodded towards the other side of the room. I followed her gaze. Sitting, or I should say slumped, on the settee in front of the bay window was another woman. The first thing to strike me was a yellow stump of bone protruding from her left leg just below the knee.

The ragged and splintered bone was smeared with blood and fatty tissue that glistened greasily under the artificial light. Her foot was attached to the ankle by what looked like skin alone. Above the knee her leg was contorted at crazy angles like an old pipe cleaner. Blood was everywhere. There were huge, deep cuts across both her thighs and her clothing hung in shreds as though someone had set about it with a Stanley knife. Her left arm was broken and twisted and through the tattered, blood-soaked clothing I could see many more lacerations, deep and open enough to clearly expose muscle and fat. Her head was thrown back, revealing deep cuts and gashes to her neck. She was breathing, or I should say snoring; a fine mist of blood was sprayed on to her chest with each exhalation. She was deeply unconscious and blood was trickling from one ear.

Even in my darkest imaginings I couldn't have dreamed up such injuries. The shock of discovering her like this in someone's living room only added to my sense of disbelief. In all probability she had a fractured

skull and her neck might be broken, along with goodness knows how many other bones. She had lost a
bucket of blood and her leg looked as though it would
fall off if it were touched. She was breathing, but for
how long? I glanced stupidly down at my first aid bag,
and then across at Howard. His face was impassive as
he returned my look and said in a calm voice, 'I'm
going to get what we need from the ambulance. In the
meantime you check her over as best you can . . . and
get some oxygen on her. All you have to remember for
the time being are the three Bs.'

The three Bs . . . I had to think. Breathing! Yes, that
was where to start: check her airway for any
obstructions. It was clear, and I inserted a Guedal
airway into her mouth to prevent her tongue falling
back, then I placed her on the maximum oxygen flow.
What next? Bleeding. I checked her over as best I could
without actually moving her. The wounds, which had
obviously been pumping out blood before we arrived,
had now started to congeal and peripheral shutdown
prevented any further blood loss. Thankfully no
arteries seemed to have been ruptured. Now what?
Bones. The blood from her ear suggested a fractured
skull. One arm and leg were shattered, but there was no
way of assessing her pelvis and ribs. Her neck was
another unknown quantity and would have to be
immobilized. The obvious violence visited on her plus
her fast, thready pulse made internal injuries likely.
How had she sustained such horrific injuries in such a

minor accident? And who on earth had brought her into the house?

I looked round to find H at my side with splints, straps, bandages, an array of cervical collars and a Scoop stretcher. He also had another ambulance crew with him. They weren't from the Street, but had happened to be passing and spotted H struggling to carry all the bits and pieces. Trouble has a tendency to find ambulance crews without them going looking for it, but on this occasion their curiosity got the better of them – luckily for us, as we were certainly going to need help getting the woman out of the house.

H took over from here on in. He'd made his own swift assessment and started by getting me to hold the woman's head steady while he fitted a rigid collar. I continued to hold her head while he directed the splinting of her leg and arm, saying that any other broken bones would have to look after themselves. There seemed to me to be too many priorities. The head injury, possible neck and spinal damage, internal haemorrhage . . . they were all priorities.

As he worked, H said, as much to himself as anybody else, 'Who in their right mind would think of bringing her into the house?'

It was the little girl from the hallway who provided the answer.

'She came through the window while we were having our tea.'

'*What?*' Even the normally imperturbable Howard was shaken.

I wasn't sure I'd heard correctly either. The girl's mother explained that our patient had been walking along the pavement when a car left the road and struck her, catapulting her into the air. Lucky might not be the right word, but she was lucky in that instead of hitting the building, she crashed through the front bay window. Her body had parted the curtains and she had landed exactly as we had found her on the settee. We hadn't noticed the broken window from the outside; it was dark and we'd had no reason to look for it. On the inside there was very little evidence of what had happened; the curtains had fallen neatly back into place, effectively hiding the shattered window frame.

It might have explained everything, but it didn't make it any easier to come to terms with such a bizarre series of events. I was still trying to take it all in as H did his final checks, and with the help of the others we manoeuvred the Scoop stretcher into position. The Scoop stretcher is an all-metal flat bed, which breaks apart down the middle to allow each side to be separately eased under the patient and then the two are clipped back together. Once the straps are securely tied and the head is taped down, the patient can be moved without risk of aggravating any injuries. It may well be the inspiration for the expression 'scoop and run' and if it is, then it's very apt. Thankfully the woman was maintaining her own airway, and when everything was ready four pairs of hands carefully eased the stretcher through the house and into the ambulance. With the 'scooping' done, it was now time to get 'running'.

The only place this poor woman's life was going to be saved was in an operating theatre, meaning that once she was safely constrained, speed became the essence. She was fortunate that the Birmingham Accident Hospital, staffed by top-class trauma experts, was relatively close by. It's difficult to estimate how long we spent in the house, but it was probably somewhere between twelve and fifteen minutes. The journey to hospital was about four, making it less than twenty minutes from innocently sauntering down the path to delivering the patient to the trauma room. Not bad.

When I eventually emerged from Casualty, the excitement and physical exertion began to take its toll and I found myself nervously puffing on a cigarette and going over and over the case in my head. Then I thought of the family in the house. I couldn't begin to imagine what it must be like for them. There they were, sitting with their evening meals on their laps and watching TV, when the bloodied body of a young woman exploded into the room and landed neatly on the sofa. Poor kids. While I was deep in thought, Howard was cleaning our equipment and tidying it away on the ambulance. It was my job, but when I went over to help he waved me away, telling me to finish my fag. He was everything I expected an ambulance man to be: cool, calm and professional throughout, quietly delivering unhurried instructions with an authority that demanded respect. He was a good bloke all right ... certainly not someone who deserved to have a dozen snooker balls dropped on his head.

When I checked on the patient's progress a couple of weeks later, it was to be told that she'd regained consciousness but had no memory of the incident. Her physical injuries were expected to heal with time. As so often happens, I lost track of her progress after that.

Chapter Eleven

If the case of the 'flying lady' taught me anything, it was that I could at least handle unpleasant sights. While this revelation came as a welcome relief, it didn't stop the memory of the poor woman's appalling injuries staying with me for a long time afterwards. And I wasn't fooled into thinking I was made of sterner stuff than anyone else, for I began to appreciate that being actively involved in a patient's treatment is a much easier option than watching passively from the sidelines.

We had no time to dwell on anything other than our responsibilities to the woman. We had to stabilize her to the best of our ability in preparation for the journey to hospital. Working to this end meant that, rather than finding her injuries repellent, we saw them as a series of problems to be resolved. Of course, having Howard calling the shots made all the difference. Forget television nurses and doctors barking orders at each other and hysterically demanding blood pressures or pulse rates – true efficiency comes with calm authority born of self-belief, qualities only gained with time and experience. H had plenty for both of us; just watching him was worth weeks in a classroom.

The 'flying lady' also gained me a certain kudos in the messroom. People who hadn't spoken a word to me since I first walked into the place would sit themselves in a chair next to mine and ask how I was settling in, then come out with something like 'I hear you had a nasty job the other day.'

I'd learned enough by now to be suitably enigmatic.

'Oh really, which job would that be?'

'You know . . . the woman who went through the window.'

'Ah, that job. Yes, it was pretty nasty . . .'

There was no fooling H though. For days afterwards I bombarded him with a string of 'what if' questions. What if she'd suddenly started to vomit blood? What if she'd gone into respiratory arrest when we tried to move her? What if she'd had a fit on the way out to the ambulance? What if she'd gone into cardiac arrest? H stuck it as long as he could before bringing it to an end in his own inimitable way.

'What if,' he asked, 'she'd suddenly sat up and started whistling "Dixie"?'

Anyone else would just have told me to shut up.

I was lucky enough to stay with H through the hectic weeks leading up to Christmas. Although the majority of 999 calls were the direct result of people drinking too much, it was a generally light-hearted period. Suitably imbued with the festive spirit, the drunks were surprisingly amiable, apologetic even, and it rubbed off on the Casualty staff, who threw a few extra smiles around and hung bits of tinsel and holly from doorframes.

The only intoxicated people I felt anything approaching sympathy for were those who'd been led astray. They were usually young and, when it came to Christmas office parties, naive to say the least. Though they were unused to downing shedloads of booze, their workmates would often coax them into imbibing far more than they could handle. What may have seemed harmless fun at the time would frequently turn into a nightmare later. One victim stands out in my memory for two reasons. First, I felt sorry for her, and secondly, it gave me an insight into student life that, for me, had so far been a closed book.

University students had hired a lush banqueting suite in which to hold their end-of-term Christmas binge. Undaunted by the grand surroundings, they set about enjoying themselves in the time-honoured way: getting as drunk as possible, as fast as possible. H had to be careful negotiating the winding drive as students in formal evening dress were meandering aimlessly about gulping in the night air, presumably in a vain effort to sober up. The lads' ties were loosened, their shirts were hanging out and their jackets had long since been discarded. The women, having fewer clothes to discard, made do by carrying their shoes and hitching up their dresses to make movement easier. Any one of them could have been our patient but with no one making an attempt to flag us down we carried on up the drive.

We were almost at the entrance and about to pass a group of three or four lads when one of them suddenly stumbled forward, clutching his chest with both hands. His legs wobbled and gave way, forcing him to his knees. He held this position for a moment before raising a faltering arm towards us in supplication. A look of agony crossed his features as he crashed face first on to the grass where he twitched a couple of times before becoming perfectly still.

'That wasn't a bad effort,' H said as he steered the ambulance round the body without slowing down.

I craned my neck to look back. 'Aren't you going to stop?'

'Stop?' H sounded puzzled.

'He's collapsed! Shouldn't we go and help?'

H smiled. 'It's something you're going to have to get used to. When youngsters have a bellyful of beer and spot an ambulance they just can't resist playing the prat. They either hold their chest and pretend to be dying or, more often than not, grab their leg and pretend it's broken. That gives them the chance to hop around a bit. I have to hand it to that lad though. He was impressive . . . Must be what a university education does for you.'

As Howard was talking, I checked the view behind in the door mirror. The lad stood up and dusted himself off.

H found somewhere to park close to the front doors and we made our way to the glass-fronted building. Waiting on the steps was a striking woman in her early thirties who, in company with the others, wore a black ankle-length evening dress. She threw us a horsy smile and launched into a jumbled explanation of why we'd been called.

'Hi, guys! Sorry about calling you out but we've got a girl who's had a bit too much to drink. I simply don't know what to do with her. I'm Penny by the way, I'm kind of in charge of this lot.' She looked warmly at the young people lurching around and carried on talking as she led us through the building, breaking off occasionally to sidestep fondling couples strewn about the floor. 'To be honest with you, she's got very drunk. I'm sure there's nothing else involved . . . no drugs or anything like that.'

When we reached the ladies' toilets she stopped and, leaning towards us, spoke in a conspiratorial voice.

'She's French, you see, and I don't think she's used to drinking so much in one evening. I know they drink a lot of wine and stuff over there but, when it comes to vodka, it was silly of her to try and keep up with our girls.' The information was passed on with a sense of pride, and as if being French and not having the ability to drink limitless quantities of alcohol was a dark secret best kept between the three of us. Her point made, she pushed open the door.

Neither Howard nor I was prepared for the cacophony of shrill female voices that suddenly assailed us. The place was bursting at the seams with young women dressed in evening gowns. Some were standing, some were sitting, but they all had two things in common: each held a glass, and each was talking at the top of her voice. Penny was already forcing her way through the mêlée, nodding and grinning in response to the shrieked greetings of the girls she squeezed past. We followed in her wake, skirting a group of four or five girls sitting round a table and swigging from a bottle of wine passing between them. When one began choking and spluttering it elicited high-pitched squeals of delight from the others and only added to my sense of incredulity.

It certainly wasn't like any toilet I'd ever known. Even through the throng, I could see it was a lovely spacious area with room enough for plenty of wicker chairs and small tables. In addition to its obvious function it had been designed as a retreat, a place where a woman could relax and gather her thoughts, or maybe exchange gossip while touching up her face. Everything, from the ornate ceiling to the heavily carpeted floor, looked expensive. Six gold-tapped washbasins ran along the wall to our right and behind these was a mirror at least twelve feet long. Subdued wall lighting reflected warmly off the deep red tiles and, standing on pedestals at each end of the mirror, potted plants cascaded greenery to ground level.

Under normal circumstances this arrangement would probably be considered subtly tasteful. But tonight could not be described as normal circumstances. Stretched out along the narrow ledge behind the basins and below the mirror was the slumbering form of an overweight girl. Like a basking seal on the shoreline she snored heavily through quivering nostrils and half-parted lips. She was oblivious to everything, including the fact that her ringlets were tumbling down into a basin where another girl, shoulders heaving, was making grotesque noises in an effort to vomit. For a moment I thought that she was our patient, but Penny pushed past without a second glance and continued to the far side of the room where the toilet cubicles were.

She stopped at the only open door and gestured inside.

'Here she is . . . This is Chantal.' Leaning her head in slightly, she shouted, 'Chantal, Chantal, wake up! There are two nice men here to help you.'

H and I peered over her shoulder, to be rewarded by a singularly distasteful sight. Chantal was sitting on the floor with her back resting against the toilet pedestal. For lateral balance her legs were splayed wide apart, each knee wedged against the partition walls on either side. The long black dress was hitched up to her thighs to reveal her tights, which were pulled halfway down her shins. Her head was slumped forward and a long, swaying strand of saliva spiralled down from her chin to merge with a substantial pool of vomit in her lap. Howard edged his way in and crouched in front of her.

'Hello, Chantal.' Getting no response, he slipped effortlessly into French. '*Bonjour*, Chantal!'

She lifted her head and blinked. '*Bonjour.*' Her skin had the pallor of a belly-up fish by moonlight. Her make-up, so carefully applied at the beginning of the evening, was smeared across her face leaving her with the look of a gargoyle. She narrowed her eyes and tried to focus on H.

'*Qui êtes-vous?*'

H, who'd just exhausted his French vocabulary, covered his confusion by taking her pulse.

Another girl appeared beside us. 'She's wrecked, you know! We're all wrecked! But she's so seriously, seriously wrecked!' She giggled, burped and, putting her hand to her mouth in mock apology, lurched on past to one of the other cubicles and started banging on the door while hopping from foot to foot. 'Judy! Judy! Are you still in there, for Christ's sake? Come on, I want a pee, I'm bloody desperate!'

The reply from behind the closed door was short and to the point.

'Get lost, will you. I'm not well!'

'I need a pee!'

'Use the bloody garden then!'

Cubicle doors banged open and closed as a constant flow of girls passed in and out. The air was filled with the sound of retching, flushing toilets, shouts, laughter and giggles. The incongruity between the way these young ladies were dressed in lovely gowns and high heels, and in the way they were behaving, made the scene all the more bizarre. I felt that I was witnessing a surreal play, and said so out loud to no one in particular.

'This is like something out of a Ken Russell film.'

Penny overheard me. 'Ken Russell? Oh yes, I see what you mean! Ken Russell. Yes, Ken Russell . . . very good!' She threw back her head and gave a laugh that might have brought the chandelier down. Turning to the room, she shouted at the top of her voice. 'Hey, everybody! Smile . . . we're in the movies!'

It was then I realized she was every bit as drunk as the girls she was supposed to be supervising.

H and I pulled on our gloves and glanced at each other as we heaved the dripping Chantal on to our carry chair, aware that we were the only sober people in the building. After wrapping her in a blanket only a tuft of hair at the top of her head was left exposed. As I looked down at her I wondered what her thoughts would have been if she'd known that by the end of the evening no one would have dared touch her unless protected by rubber gloves. A small, muffled voice came from under the blanket.

'*Où est-ce qu'on va?*'

I looked at the tuft of hair and said, '*Hôpital*, Chantal. *Hôpital*.'

Chantal doubtless learned her lesson, but for some it was way too late to talk about learning lessons. Only a few days later Howard and I were called to a tower block in Nechells, which at the time was a horribly deprived area of inner Birmingham. We foolishly took the lift and ended up counting off every second as it rattled and banged its way up to the tenth floor. The flat we were looking for was just across the landing. After knocking on the open door without getting a reply, we made our way tentatively down the hall to the living room. The cloying atmosphere was as depressing as it was familiar. Bottles, cans, cigarette ends and chip wrappers littered the floor, while above our heads the light from a sixty-watt bulb grudgingly cast a greasy glow over the room. Two battered settees and a couple of armchairs were occupied by the shadowy figures of several middle-aged men. What air there was must have been recycled between them so many times that it was a wonder the wall-mounted gas fire could find the oxygen to keep burning. We'd been warned beforehand to be careful because the place had been taken over as a squat, but as I looked around it was clear there was no threat here.

Not wishing to venture too far inside, I stopped and made our presence known.

'Hello . . . someone called for us?'

A grunt came from the shadows. 'Come in.'

I didn't notice a bottle of cider lying on the floor until my foot inadvertently sent it rolling into the room, where it came to rest at the feet of a bearded man on the settee. He stared down at it as the contents sloshed back and forth then slowly lifted his eyes to me. A large pitted nose and two rheumy eyes were the only features visible through the wild hair and beard. I think he tried to smile.

'Hello, pal. You the ambulance?' He shifted in his chair in preparation for getting to his feet but after one aborted attempt he wisely decided to stay put. 'Thanks for coming. It's young Jason. He needs to go to hospital . . . he's bad.'

I looked around. Five dishevelled men were slumped in the various seats. I didn't know if they were drunk or drugged but, to a man, they all looked battered, worn out and ill.

'Which one's Jason?' I asked.

The greybeard gestured languidly towards a nearby armchair where a man sat staring at the floor.

'That's him, that's Jason.'

I walked over and looked down at the top of his head. 'Jason?'

'Yeah.'

'What's the problem?'

'Nothing, mate, I'm fine. There's nothing wrong with me. I don't know what they're making all the fuss about.'

'There must be something wrong,' I said. 'Your

mates wouldn't have called an ambulance for nothing, would they?'

I waited for him to say something. When he continued staring at the floor without replying, I tried again.

'Please look at me, Jason. I'm trying to talk to you.'

Again he didn't reply, and I cast a questioning glance at the greybeard, who said, 'Don't waste your time trying to talk, mate, just take him away.'

'I can't drag someone to hospital if they don't want to go,' I said. 'Anyway, I don't even know what's supposed to be wrong with him.'

'He's coughing up blood. Just look at the state of him, he's at death's door.'

A chorus of mumbled agreement came from the shadows.

I crouched down to Jason's level and spoke to him again.

'Come on, I can't go away until you speak to me properly. We've got to get to the bottom of this.'

When he reluctantly raised his head I was shocked to see he was younger than me. I'd assumed him to be in his forties, but now it was clear that he couldn't be more than twenty. He was grimy, his hair lank and greasy, but through this shone a good-natured and intelligent face. What was he doing here among these broken-down middle-aged alcoholics?

'There's nothing wrong with me,' he said softly. 'You shouldn't be wasting your time here. You must have better things to do.'

'He's been bringing up blood for the last two days,' slurred a voice behind me.

'Is that right?' I asked. 'Have you been bringing up blood, Jason?'

'Only a bit, I'll be OK. I'm not going to hospital.'

I felt his pulse. It was fast and thready. He looked ill.

'Jason,' I said, 'this could be serious. You really must come and get checked over—'

He cut across me. 'Please . . . I don't want to be rude, I appreciate that you're trying to help, but please, leave me alone. I'm not going anywhere and that's the end of it.'

From the tone of his voice I knew we weren't going to change his mind, but none the less I went through a routine of persuasion I hoped would work. It was futile. He was apologetic but adamant; the thought of hospital obviously terrified him. I let Howard take over in the hope he might get through to him.

I moved to the window and stared out through the brittle net curtains. It was obvious Jason had no intention of leaving the flat and being parted from his alcohol, drugs, glue or whatever it was he'd become dependent on. What a waste. How could someone so young become little more than a piece of human flotsam drifting between filthy squats? Ten floors below, the city spread into the distance like a vast illuminated carpet and, as I listened to Howard's fatherly tone trying to cajole Jason into coming with us, it struck me that he was indeed someone's son. Perhaps down there somewhere, among the myriad of lights, or in a town or village a hundred miles away, a family waited anxiously for news of him.

Howard eventually gave up trying to coax him. There was nothing left for us to do. Seeing us ready to leave, Jason's bearded friend managed to heave himself unsteadily to his feet and stood in front of me while he searched through his fogged brain for the right words.

'Look, pal . . . Jason's been like a son to me since he's been here . . . You've got to do something to help him. You can't just walk away.'

I felt guilty, and spoke without much conviction. 'We've done our best to persuade him. You can see for yourself that he won't come with us. All I can do is to try and get a doctor to come out and see him.'

The man looked confused and angry.

'This is a squat. No doctor will come out to us. Drag him into the ambulance. We'll help you, won't we, lads?' He turned to the others for support but they only shifted in their seats and said nothing.

'I can't do that!' I raised my voice slightly to make my point. 'He's conscious, he's rational . . . I can't drag him into the ambulance against his will. It's against the law.'

The bearded man ran a hand across his face and slumped back into the chair, from where he scooped up the bottle of cider from the floor in one fluid movement. After a long swig he belched, and made his feelings clear.

'The law's a load of bollocks!'

At the door I turned to ask Jason one last time if he would come with us. He was staring at me, looking steadily into my eyes with a gaze I found unnerving. It didn't convey any appeal for help or sympathy; it was more a look of mild surprise that anyone outside this room should care about him. He was grateful, grateful to me when I'd done nothing. I felt strangely affected. Howard spoke for me.

'Are you sure you won't come with us, Jason?'

The reply came without hesitation. 'No thanks. Really, I'll be all right.'

'Promise me you'll go and see a doctor in the morning,' I said.

He smiled back, relieved that the pressure was off. 'Yes, yes, I'll do that.'

I knew he wouldn't.

The incident faded from my mind until three days later when a crew came on to station grumbling that dropping a body off at the mortuary wasn't a good way to start Christmas Eve. Only half listening behind my newspaper, I picked up the gist of their conversation. They'd found the body of a scruffy young man at dawn in a quiet side street. He was curled up in a doorway and in the early morning light they'd assumed he was asleep, but when they reached him it was clear he'd been dead for a few hours. He'd died alone. Whoever called 999 hadn't seen fit to wait. It wasn't an uncommon tale, but my interest was roused when one of them said, 'No great loss, I suppose. Only a druggy living in a Nechells squat.'

I put down my newspaper. 'You say he was a young bloke?'

'Yeah, early twenties. Why?'

I tried to sound casual. 'His name wasn't Jason, was it?'

'Yes, I think it was.' He reached for his notebook. 'That's it, Jason Hughes. He had the address of a squat in Nechells in his pocket.' He put the book away and looked at me curiously. 'You didn't know him, did you?'

Did I know him? 'No,' I said. 'Not really.'

Chapter Twelve

Finding my name on the New Year's Eve rota these days doesn't exactly fill me with joy. It's a bit like parachuting; one jump is enough to make you realize you never want to do it again. But without the benefit of experience, in 1977 I was actually looking forward to my first New Year's Eve on duty. I knew it would be a mad, hectic night of partygoers but, in my naivety, I expected a general air of goodwill to win through. How wrong I was. Not only did the shift severely dent my youthful illusions; it proved to be the harbinger of every New Year to come.

I know most people have a good time; our problem is that we only get to meet the people who are having a bad time. A combination of booze, excitement, fragile emotions and failed expectations brings out the worst in some people, and it's the same every year. Recently, after yet another *Groundhog Day* experience, I scribbled down a few notes after each case and later transcribed the whole shambles in detail. What follows describes that particular night, and I've no doubt it will ring a bell with any ambulance crew in any other city across the country:

11.05 p.m.
The first case Paul and I were given seemed designed to get us in the mood for the night to come. Waiting for us out on the street was a dumpy, nervous young woman. Her name was Julie and she described herself as the patient's ex-girlfriend. We followed her into the building and on our way up to the third floor Paul asked what the problem was.

'It's all my fault. If I hadn't come round to see him none of this would have happened. Ian and I broke up recently, but I thought it might be friendly just to pop in and wish him a happy new year for old times' sake. He was pretty miserable, and got worse when I told him I had to go. He gets emotional at the best of times and when I made it clear I wasn't staying he went into the kitchen and poured a load of bleach into a glass of vodka.'

'He didn't drink it, did he?' Paul asked.

'No, but he said he was going to. I tried to get it off him but he went into the toilet and locked the door. Then I called you.'

All was quiet in the flat when Paul tapped on the bathroom door.

'Hello, Ian. It's the ambulance service.'

163

There was a pause before Ian reacted.

'What the hell do you want?'

'Julie's called us. Can you come out and talk to us?'

'Who do you think you are? You can't barge into my flat and tell me what to do!'

'I haven't barged in, and I'm not telling you what to do.' Paul's tone was friendly and reasoned. 'Come on, I feel silly talking through a door like this.'

'Go away then.'

'We can't go away. Julie says you've threatened to drink some bleach. We're worried about you.'

'Worried about me? You're only here because you're paid to be.'

This was undeniably true, but Paul denied it all the same. 'That's ridiculous. We're here because we want to help.'

'Don't make me laugh. You don't know me. Why the hell should you care about me? I don't care about you.'

Good question. Paul tried to deflect it. 'Your girlfriend cares.'

'She isn't my girlfriend. She's dumped me!'

True again. While Paul tried to think of a suitable reply, Ian continued.

'She only came round to rub it in. She's got her whole night planned out . . . and it doesn't include me.'

Paul then came up with what I thought was a bit of indisputable logic. 'She wouldn't be here if she didn't care about you, would she?'

'If she cared about me, why would she dump me?'

I don't think Paul was keen to go down this path, so he tried a different tack. 'There's no point locking yourself in the toilet. You can still enjoy New Year's Eve if nothing else.'

There was a pause, which gave me hope a chord might have been struck. I was wrong.

Ian was too incredulous to respond immediately. When he did, there was an aggressive edge to his voice. 'You havin' a laugh?'

'No . . . I'm just trying to say . . .'

I think it fair to say that as far as his negotiating skills were concerned, Paul would make a good car-park attendant.

And so it went on for the next fifteen minutes. Eventually, with the situation deadlocked, I whispered to Paul that the only option left was to put the door in. After all, it was only a flimsy bolt and we would be in before Ian could put the glass to his lips. It wasn't as if he had a gun or anything. Julie overheard and agreed, but threw in a word of warning.

'You'll have to be careful when you get inside. He's got a switchblade. He cut his neck with it earlier.'

It's funny how often this kind of thing happens. You think you've gathered all the facts and are ready to make a decision, then a bit more information gets casually drip-fed into the scenario. Paul looked at her, mystified.

'Why didn't you tell us that before?'

'I thought you knew.'

'How could we . . . ?'

There wasn't any point continuing down this line. Things had changed. We had cornered an unbalanced person with a knife in one hand and a glass of bleach in the other. He was threatening to use them on himself, but how were we to know he wouldn't turn homicidal? I didn't fancy getting drenched in bleach and simultaneously stabbed. The *Evening News* headline would write itself: 'MERCY-DASH HEROES DENIED MERCY IN NEW YEAR'S EVE BLOODBATH Full details on page three.'

By one of those strange coincidences that happen now and again, four hefty police officers appeared unbidden at the door while I was trying to figure out how to switch on the mobile phone to call them. The heftiest, and the leader by the look of it, was a WPC. She listened as Paul brought her up to speed and then turned to face the locked door. Using a saccharine voice dripping every platitude that sprang to mind, she started to work on Ian. Ten frustrating minutes later, her tone had upped a few octaves and assumed a dangerous pitch.

Five minutes later she was barking at him to stand back because she was going to break the door down (a task for which she wouldn't need any help). I noticed her colleagues checking their canisters of mace spray. Having been on the wrong end of that stuff once before, I knew it feels as if someone's thrown an ant's nest into your face and I moved a bit further down the hall. The WPC snapped open her steel truncheon and pointed out loudly to Ian that he would be the one paying for the repairs.

After all our efforts to cajole and persuade, it was this throwaway comment that hit home. Ian was alarmed.

'Hang on, you can't do that!'

The WPC's jaw tightened. 'Can't I? Just bloody watch!'

'No! I mean . . . don't break the door. I'll open it.'

As he spoke there was the sound of a bolt being drawn. The WPC quickly moved forward and, grasping the handle, held the door shut while addressing Ian in a frighteningly commanding manner.

'Drop the knife on the floor!' There was an immediate clatter in response.

'Now,' she said, 'kick it away from you.' There was the sound of steel slithering on lino.

'Where's the bleach?'

'On the floor.'

'It better be!' With that she pushed open the door and piled in.

Ian was on the floor with one arm draped over the closed toilet seat. He didn't measure up to anyone's idea of a homicidal maniac. He was about twenty-five, diminutive and – I hate to use the expression 'nerdish' but, as it fits, I will. Beside him was the glass containing the noxious brew of bleach and vodka and in the corner lay not a switchblade but a Stanley knife. From my position peering over the WPC's shoulder I could see the cut on his neck was nothing more than a minor scratch. The policewoman felt it safe to return to a more motherly tone.

'Come on then, Ian, let's get you out of here.'

It didn't prove that easy. He seemed quite attached to the toilet and, seeing he had a captive audience, used the opportunity to have his say about what was wrong with the world and everybody in it.

When he reluctantly emerged into the hall he was still in a defiant mood, and I found myself silently agreeing with him again when he questioned the point of going to hospital.

'They'll just stick me in the waiting room for hours.'

'No, they won't.' I tried to be convincing. 'There will be someone to talk over your problems with and offer help if you need it.'

'Yeah, like giving me an appointment to see a shrink next October.'

I felt he was being a little optimistic on that one, but pointed out there might be a drug regime that would help him.

'Fill me with pills! You're just like all the rest. Stop pretending you care, will you! I don't care about you . . . and you don't care about me. Yeah? You got that?'

'It doesn't have to be that way. We can talk this through.'

'You're talking garbage and you know it.'

He must have been a mind reader, or maybe I just have an honest face.

We eventually dropped him off at the hospital and before booking clear I looked at my watch. It was five to twelve. Just before midnight is a bit like the eye of the storm, nice while it lasts but you know what's coming. When midnight struck, fireworks burst all over the sky and some DJ ranted hysterically on the radio. I exchanged a lacklustre handshake with Paul. A few minutes later we pulled into the Street and walked through to the messroom where I took my coat off, sat down and, in the same movement, got up to answer the phone.

12.10 a.m.

'You've only called to wish us a happy new year, haven't you?' I asked before the other person had a chance to speak.

'No,' replied a female voice, 'I've called to send you on a 999 for a man with a blister on his buttock.'

'What?' I was ready for virtually anything, but this came as a surprise.

'It's a disgrace, isn't it?' the girl continued. 'The phones are starting to go mad and I have to send you on something like this.'

Surely there was more to it?

'Is it an old person?' I asked.

'Nope. He's thirty-two, and his GP's been treating the problem for a couple of weeks. He says the doctor told him that if it didn't improve he should go to the hospital.'

'He couldn't have meant by ambulance at this time of night. Is the bloke drunk?'

'No, I don't think so. Oh, happy new year, by the way.'

We had to drive two miles to pick this character up and take him the half-mile or so to hospital. He had a small area on his buttock resembling a pressure sore. There was no blister or seepage and otherwise he was a fit, healthy individual who could just as easily have walked out to a taxi as he walked out to the ambulance. There is, of course, a fundamental difference between ambulances and taxis. Ambulances are free and, what's more, the government demands they reach the 'patient' within fourteen minutes. For the life of me, I can't understand why the taxi drivers' union isn't up in arms; they should start lobbying Parliament on the grounds of unfair competition.

With his personal details, medical history and vital signs duly recorded in A3 duplicate, we dropped him off at the hospital and watched as he made his way to the Casualty waiting area. If he was hoping to beat the queue by arriving in an ambulance, he was in for a rude awakening. The waiting time posted on the moving LED screen for non-urgent cases was something like four hours and rising. I took a smidgen of comfort from this as I sipped a coffee and idly watched a procession of people with one minor injury after another stagger through the

Casualty doors. Drunk, as most of them were, they wouldn't have been half as bad if they were on their own. It's the two or three rowdy mates in tow who invariably cause the trouble. There must be an agency somewhere so you can hire objectionable individuals to accompany you when you know you'll be sitting around in Casualty for hours, an organization set up in opposition to the hospital visitors' scheme.

12.50 a.m.
After draining our coffee, we made our way outside to find the temperature had dropped and the steady rain that had been falling all night had turned into a lashing downpour. Six ambulances were parked in the bay and, with our anoraks pulled up over our heads, we made a dash for the one we hoped was ours. The radio traffic was incessant and within seconds of booking clear we were off on another job. 'Man collapsed in the street.' Here was something novel on New Year's Day. Listening to the rain hammering against the windscreen I was confident that by the time we got there he would be up and gone. It simply wasn't the kind of night to lie about outside.

A few minutes later I was proved wrong. Our head-lights picked him out on the pavement, looking like a bundle of rags washed up by the tide. A concerned motorist had stopped to help him and, finding him barely rousable, made the 999 call. Despite his umbrella, the Good Samaritan was drenched and grabbed the chance to make a quick getaway while Paul and I checked the patient over. Not finding any sign of physical injuries, we heaved him on to the stretcher and into the warmth of the ambulance.

Once on board we were able to get a better look at him. He was pretty groggy, but otherwise the only obvious abnormality was his temperature. It was about two degrees below normal, which wasn't surprising as he was soaking wet and had probably been lying on the pavement for some time. He was verbally aggressive when I persisted in pressing a biro into the cuticle of one of his fingers in an attempt to gauge his response to pain, and then dropped back off to sleep.

Mindful that it's my duty not to prejudge a situation, I carefully considered the possibilities. He might be a diabetic. A quick test of his sugar levels ruled that one out. He might have suffered a stroke. He had full limb movement and his verbal skills were such that he was able to tell me to fuck off, so a stroke was unlikely. He might have suffered a head injury. There was no evidence to support that. This left another possibility, the one I favoured: he might just be pissed. His breath smelled as if his stomach had been used as a fermentation tank, and the liberal supply of vomit on his chest, rain-diluted as it was, was probably about 100 per cent proof. Not that I am one to prejudge, you understand. He got all the care and attention he deserved but, despite the rain, I had to open the windows and skylight when it became apparent that, apart from being incontinent of urine, he'd also filled his pants.

The hospital waiting area had come to resemble Digbeth coach station on a bank holiday Monday. Most people, although loud, were reasonably good-natured and happy to pass the time exchanging drunken anecdotes while they compared wounds. There was a minority who kept the security staff on their toes, but they soon found themselves being escorted out into the rain. As we jostled our way towards triage I noticed the man with the sore buttock sitting uncomfortably amid the mayhem. He was fending off a couple of young girls in full Goth gear who seemed determined he should take a swig from the can of lager being waved under his nose. He wore the look of someone who knew he'd made a big mistake. Good.

The corridor leading to the triage area was filled with ambulance crews waiting in line to hand over their motley collection of patients to the nurse. Her un-enviable task was to categorize each one in order of importance as they arrived: no easy job when virtually everyone wheeled in front of her was befuddled by drink. We do have some say in this process. When we feel our patient needs immediate attention it's up to us to make our way to the front and state our case. In view of the fact that our man was doubly incontinent, semi-conscious and hovering on the edge of hypothermia, I felt I had no choice but to speak up on his behalf. As a result we jumped the queue and were back out on the corridor with an empty stretcher in a matter of minutes.

Paul went off to fetch the coffee and I began to think about food. We knew before starting the shift that there was about as much chance of being offered a meal break as being wished a happy new year, so we had come prepared. Any food we brought in had to be eaten 'on the hoof' and, with this in mind, Marie had carefully selected my nibbles from the Marks & Spencer food hall the previous afternoon. There was a posh pork pie, cold chicken-tikka slices, dried German sausage, ham off the bone in sandwiches and, to finish, a fruit-laden cream trifle.

Back in the ambulance I opened my little hamper and surveyed the contents. Lying between the pork pie and the chicken, and looking about as appetizing as a mummified penis, was the German sausage. I've read somewhere that U-boat crews more or less lived on these wretched things during the war; well, they must have been tough guys. It would have to wait. The chicken tikka was another matter – it was asking to be eaten, and I got stuck in while listening to Control pleading over the radio for any available ambulances to come forward and claim one of the many outstanding 999 cases. They reeled off a list of locations, presumably in the hope we might be tempted. Eventually my conscience got the better of me and I jabbed a yellow-stained finger at the 'clear' button on the console. Our reward was a trip to a small nightclub in the city centre where a woman had apparently collapsed.

1.40 a.m.

Birmingham is a city that can't leave itself alone. At the time of writing it's going through yet another of its protracted redevelopment phases. For redevelopment, read bulldoze everything in sight and then rebuild. Buildings disappear overnight, one-way streets are reversed, roads vanish, and underpasses that cost a fortune to excavate thirty years ago are filled in. New roads, roundabouts and offices, albeit in slightly different positions, appear in their place. A city I used to know like the back of my hand has become an alien environment, which is a long-winded way of explaining why we had to go round the new one-way system twice before finding the club.

It was the kind of place you could easily miss, but there was no missing the large West Indian doorman standing on the pavement holding out his arm as if flagging down a cab. He showed us into the foyer, where our patient was sitting on a chair looking limp and bedraggled. She'd collapsed inside the club and been led out for some fresh air. Since then she'd sat staring at the floor, making no attempt to move or talk. Her husband had disappeared and the bouncer didn't know what to do, until he came up with the idea of packing her off in an ambulance.

We did our best to interrogate the woman but received only monosyllabic replies (the general thrust of which was for us to go away). We were still trying to get through to her when the interior door to the club opened and a young woman tottered unsteadily over to us.

'I'm her friend,' she said. 'I don't know why you were called. There's nothing wrong with her.'

Paul looked doubtful. 'She doesn't look very well to me.'

'She's not drunk if that's what you're saying!'

'Nobody said she was drunk,' Paul said indignantly. Then, after a suitable pause, he asked, 'How much has she had to drink?'

The woman took a pull on her cigarette. 'Same as me.'

I looked at her and, not for the first time, wondered why some people can't just answer a question.

'How much have you had then?' Paul asked patiently.

'It's the anti-depressants she's on. They react with wine and make her go all funny.'

'Anti-depressants? Do you know how many she's taken?'

'Her husband's gone to get the car.'

Paul looked bemused but returned to the subject. 'Has she taken more than the normal dose?'

'Here he is now.' The woman was on her toes looking out of the window.

A Jaguar had pulled up in front of our ambulance and a burly middle-aged man got out of the driver's seat and dodged through the rain to the club entrance.

'Thanks, lads. I'm her husband. I'll look after her now.'

Without waiting for a response he took her by the arm and, helped by the woman friend, half dragged, half carried her to the car with an efficiency that could only have been acquired with practice.

'Hang on,' I said, 'we haven't finished talking to her. She might have changed her mind about going to hospital.'

He looked down at her. 'Do you want to go to hospital, love?'

'No, I want to go home . . . I want to go to bed.'

'There you go,' said the husband and, giving us a 'mind your own business' look, he added, 'is that good enough for you?'

There was a slamming of doors and the car, its hazard lights still flashing, drove down the road and round the corner.

We were left scratching our heads, wondering if we had just witnessed a kidnap. If she had been abducted we would doubtless read about it soon enough in the *Evening Mail*. So it was back through the rain to the ambulance, where Paul started filling out another A3 duplicate form while I took the opportunity to delve into my hamper again. The sausage looked even less attractive than earlier. Little beads of moisture had broken out all over its gnarled skin, making it look like a stick of gelignite about to go critical. Giving it a wide berth I plucked out the ham sandwich, and had just closed my mouth on it when I became aware of a face hovering by my window. What now? Couldn't I even eat a sandwich in peace? Swallowing the half-chewed mouthful, I wound down the window a few inches and didn't make a very good job of trying to sound amiable.

'Yes, can I help you?'

'Coffee? I thought you might like some coffee.'

It was the bouncer. He'd braved the rain to bring us two cups of freshly percolated coffee, bless him.

2.15 a.m.

We drank the coffee and nibbled on our food while the windows steamed up around us. It was difficult to block out the constant background chatter of the ambulance radio and after a few minutes we felt obliged to rejoin the fray. Paul booked us clear while I took the cups back. I returned to the news that we were going to a party. I looked at the address on the screen and sighed. Not one of the more fashionable districts. Baseball caps mandatory, Nike tracksuit bottoms optional . . . bring your own glue and Ecstasy tabs. With no sense of anticipation I scrolled further down the screen to find out what had prompted this last-minute invitation, and there it was: someone had been assaulted. Well, well. I put the ambulance in gear and, without the aid of a compass, found my way out of the city centre.

The street in question winds its way down quite a steep hill, lined on both sides by modest terraced housing built in the twenties to accommodate workers from the huge Dunlop plant nearby. When it and other local factories closed, the area gradually fell into decline and became something of a dumping ground for problem families displaced when their tower blocks were blown up. (Part of the council's destroy and rebuild ethos, I should hasten to add.) There's still a sprinkling of the original inhabitants left in the street, but they are pensioners now and have little choice but to live with the barbarians at their gates. From the top of the hill we could see fireworks detonating further down the road. I say detonating because they weren't the colourful sparkly things I remember seeing as a child. They were more like short-range battlefield mortars and left screaming trails capable of waking the dead. They would go roughly upwards for about thirty feet before exploding with a resounding bang that echoed across the rooftops.

There was no doubt in our minds that the source of this cacophony would prove to be our destination. I had to approach slowly as people had spilled out from the house to use the street as a launch pad for their aerial bombs. One youth caught my eye straight away. It wasn't so much his appearance – like all the others he was dressed in the obligatory tracksuit bottoms, anorak and baseball cap – it was the way he moved towards the house next door that caught my attention. His furtive, crouched, rolling gait put me in mind of a safari park ape creeping up on a car, bent on mischief.

He moved closer to the dividing wall between the two houses and lobbed a hissing firework under the next-door neighbour's bay window. It exploded immediately, triggering the youth to leap to his full height and dance about stiff-armed and stiff-legged on the balls of his feet, a look of orgasmic joy on his face. I hoped the neighbours had been sensible enough to take refuge in the back bedroom for the night.

Nobody else paid him any attention. In fact nobody paid us any attention as we made our way to the front gate and waited uncomfortably for someone to approach us. Nobody did. In the end Paul stopped one of the yobs.

'Excuse me, someone's been hurt apparently. Do you know where he is?'

The youth looked at him from bleary eyes and considered the question for some time before replying.

'No.'

'Could you ask around for us . . . maybe see if you can find him?'

'What's his name?'

'I don't know what his name is!' Paul bit his tongue. 'All I know is that someone's supposed to have been assaulted, and someone's called an ambulance.'

'Wasn't me, I haven't called no fuckin' ambulance.'

'I didn't say you had . . .' Paul gave up and looked round for someone else to ask just as a couple more lads idled up. One of them took a swig from his can and chipped in.

'Someone's takin' the piss if you ask me, mate.'

'I dare say,' Paul said wearily. 'But could you do us a favour and check inside and see if anyone needs us, please?' Neither of us fancied going into the house. There was an ugly feel about these people and their party. It was no celebration: the night was just an excuse for boorish behaviour, getting drunk, or high, or all three.

'Yeah, sure, no probs.' He staggered off into the wall of music blaring from the house, and that was the last we saw of him.

After a few minutes it dawned on us that he wasn't coming back. In the meantime we'd grown increasingly uncomfortable under the baleful gaze of the youths as they came and went. One of them, a bit older than the rest, came over to us.

'I don't know why you two are still hanging around, nobody needs you. Ain't you got nothing better to do?'

That was enough for us. It was time to leave. As we drove away, a rocket streaked past the side of the ambulance and on into someone's front garden. Paul had been looking back through the door mirror and was adamant that it had been aimed at us.

I parked up round the corner and sat back while Paul filled out another A3 duplicate report form. We normally swap seats after each job, but if the patient doesn't travel we stay as we are. This meant that Paul was getting more than his fair share of paperwork but, as they say, it's an ill wind that blows no good. I could relax. When he finished he leaned forward, pressed the 'clear' button, then sat with a fresh form on his lap ready for the next case. It wasn't long in coming. A girl was reportedly having a fit at an address half a mile away. While Paul scribbled down the details I set off for the street of terraced houses with the feeling that we were going from the frying pan into the fire.

2.50 a.m.

A fat woman of about twenty-five was waiting for us on the doorstep. She stood, hands on hips, her naked belly bulging out alarmingly from a ridiculously tight T-shirt. Two vast thighs made a brief appearance below her miniskirt before disappearing into knee-high boots. It was either a case of her being gloriously uninhibited or she wasn't one for lingering too long in front of mirrors. Her lower lip was thrust forward belligerently as we approached. She started by asking us where we thought we had been and, before we could answer, pointed out that her friend could have died twice over in the time it had taken us. Once satisfied we'd got the message, she led us through a living room strewn with cans and bottles towards the stairs. Swaying danger-ously in her high-heeled boots, and revealing a pair of buttocks that would have put a shire horse to shame, she made her way up to the first floor with Paul and me bringing up the rear. One false move on her part and the consequences for us didn't bear thinking about. On the way up she described how her friend had collapsed and had a fit. What she didn't mention was that there had been an almighty row in the house beforehand.

Our patient was lying on her back in the middle of the landing pretending to be unconscious. She could only have been seventeen or eighteen and, by the look of her, she had several hours of partying under her belt. Her eyes were puffy, her hair was a tangle and her make-up was smudged and faded. Standing beside her was a morose man of about twenty-five. He didn't acknowledge our arrival other than by moving aside slightly to let Paul have access to the girl. While Paul went through his checks I tried to get some background information from the fat girl.

It appeared that, for no apparent reason, the patient had fallen to the floor where she writhed violently for thirty seconds before drifting off into unconsciousness. I asked if she was known to be epileptic, and the answer was no. Had she been complaining of feeling ill? No. How much had she had to drink? Loads. We were interrupted by a shout from the 'unconscious' girl on the floor.

'Gerroff, you bastard!'

'Open your eyes and talk to me.' Paul had obviously applied some painful stimuli to test her consciousness level. Her eyes were open and glaring at him.

'Piss off! Nobody asked you to come.'

'Yes, they did. Your friends called us. Now sit up properly and talk to us because we're not going any-where until you do.'

She grudgingly propped herself up against the wall and adopted a sulky look before asking her friend for a fag. Paul didn't protest; there wasn't any point. She sucked greedily on the cigarette and blew a plume of smoke into the air before returning her attention to Paul.

'I'm OK. You can go.'

The fat girl interjected. 'Excuse me! You're not OK. You're going to hospital!'

'No, I'm not!'

'Yes, you are! Your eyes went all diluted, didn't they, Carl?'

Carl thought about it. 'Yeah, I suppose they were a bit diluted.'

'I'm not going nowhere, leave me alone.' She got unsteadily to her feet and, bumping off a couple of walls, made her way into the bedroom and flopped down on the bed. It was as we followed her in that I noticed smashed glass all over the floor and looked round for the source.

The bedroom door had, or, I should say, had had, a large pane of frosted glass taking up the centre section. Shards were still attached to the frame but the bulk of it was missing.

'What's been going on?' I asked the fat girl.

'Nothing.'

'Nothing? What's happened to the door? Has there been a fight?'

'No! It got broke when Carl tried to get in. Yvonne

locked herself in the bedroom and he pushed a bit too hard, that's all.'

So there had been a big argument. Carl had smashed through the door and the girl, probably frightened half to death and unable to defend herself, played the only card she had . . . to collapse and pass out. She probably threw in the 'fit' for authenticity's sake. I looked at Carl, and got back a look that I didn't much care for.

Paul wanted to wrap things up. Even though it was pretty clear what had gone on, and the 'patient' wasn't showing any of the signs you might expect to see in someone coming round from a fit, he again offered to take her to hospital for a check-up.

'No way!' Yvonne said emphatically.

Carl felt moved to speak for a second time. 'Stop pissing about! You're going, and that's it!'

'She doesn't need you to tell her what to do,' the fat girl chipped in. 'This is all your fault anyway.'

'Will you all just piss off!' Yvonne had got off the bed and was crunching barefoot over the glass back towards the landing. 'You make me sick, the pair of you.'

'Now hang on, young lady.' Clearly affronted, the fat girl followed her out. 'Who the fuck do you think you're talking to?'

Yvonne made it clear that she knew exactly who she was talking to and, in the process, triggered a slanging match between the three of them. It swung to and fro; one minute Carl and the fat girl were haranguing

Yvonne, then, for no obvious reason, Carl and Yvonne were having a go at the fat girl. When the girls eventually joined forces and turned on Carl he didn't stand much of a chance. To find yourself in the sights of two aggressively drunken women can't be much fun. When they had him backing into a corner Paul and I decided it was time to make ourselves scarce.

'We'll be off then.' Paul had raised his voice slightly. 'We're leaving the building . . . Happy new year.'

If they heard him, they chose to ignore him. We closed the door on the way out.

3.35 a.m.
Back in the ambulance, Paul started on the paperwork while I leaned back and closed my eyes. I must have drifted slightly, as the next thing I knew was Paul taking down another case. A sixty-two-year-old woman had taken an overdose. How is it they always know the age of the patient? No matter how scant the details may be of injury or location, Control can always be relied on to know the patient's exact age. A few minutes later we pulled up in front of the house. A light was burning in the living room and through the lace curtains we could see a woman sitting in an armchair. Paul rang the doorbell and waited. After a few moments the hall light came on and a woman's voice addressed us through the door.

'Who is it?'

Paul looked skyward. 'She dials 999 in the middle of

the night, we arrive five minutes later and she wants to know who it is . . . Give me strength.'

I spoke through the letterbox. 'It's the ambulance.'

'What do you want?'

Paul stared at the door. 'What do we want? You called for an ambulance, didn't you?'

'No.'

'Has anybody else in the house called for us?'

'No.'

We looked at each other. Surely we weren't at the wrong address? Why would she be sitting up on her own at this time of night? And oddly enough, from the brief glimpse we'd had of her, she did look remarkably like a sixty-two-year-old.

'Sorry to have bothered you, love.' Paul tried to sound contrite.

'That's all right.'

The light went off in the hall, and we returned to the ambulance.

Paul picked up the radio mike and explained the situation to Control. While we waited for a response, I flipped open my sandwich box and lifted out the German sausage. I rolled it cautiously between my fingers. It wasn't sweating any more. The skin, if you didn't count the odd greasy nodule, had reverted to its natural leathery state of mummification. I dropped it back in the box and took out the last of the pork pie. I listened to what Control had to say as I chewed.

We were definitely at the correct address. The

woman's name was Mrs Spencer and her son's name was Neil. Paul let out a snort.

'What on earth's her son's name got to do with anything?'

The call hadn't come from the address in question. It had been made by what Control like to describe as a 'third-party caller'. It had started when the woman phoned her son and told him she'd taken some tablets. (He also suspected there was drink involved.) Worried, he called the police, who passed it on to the ambulance service, who in turn dispatched us without a word of explanation.

'Does the woman know an ambulance was requested?' Paul asked.

'Not as far as we know.' A note of irritation had entered the controller's voice. 'We'll get the police to come and sort it out.'

Paul looked at me. 'Can you believe it? They knew the whole story, and not a bloody word to us.'

'They told us how old she was,' I pointed out through a mouthful of crumbs.

Paul drummed his fingers on the dash and came to a decision.

'I'm not sitting here like a lemon waiting for the police. Now we know what's been going on, let's go and speak to her again.'

We returned to the house and after ringing the bell Paul continued the conversation through the letterbox.

'Is that Mrs Spencer?'

'Yes.'

'It's the ambulance crew again. Neil seems to be worried about you.' Paul was trying to be pleasant.

'Is he now? Well, you can tell him I'm fine, thank you.'

'Can we come in and speak to you properly?'

'Why?'

'Just to put Neil's mind at rest, that's all.'

'Have you spoken to him?'

'Er, not as such. Look, can we come in? It's cold out here.'

To our surprise the door opened and we stepped inside.

She was a small, frail-looking woman but closer inspection revealed a hard edge to her mouth and eyes. When she spoke there was the telltale whiff of alcohol.

'Neil's worried about me, is he? New Year's Eve and no visit, not even so much as a phone call, and suddenly he's worried about me. You'd better come through.'

She tottered down the hall to the living room, where she sat down in her armchair with a sigh. The television was on but the sound was on mute. By the side of her chair were two empty wine bottles.

'So what's he been telling you?'

'We heard that you might have taken some tablets,' Paul said.

'What? An overdose, you mean?'

'Yeah, something like that.' Paul looked uncomfortable. 'Have you taken an overdose?'

'Of course not! All I've had is a glass of wine.'

'Neil says you phoned him and said you'd taken an overdose.' Paul wasn't finding it easy to suggest she was lying.

'All I said to him was that I *might* take an overdose, I didn't say I *had* taken one. God knows though, I've plenty of reason to.'

She leaned unsteadily over the side of the chair and picked up one of the bottles, but let it fall back to the floor when she saw it was empty. Paul persisted.

'Do you have any medicines in the house?'

'Yes, they're in the kitchen by the drainer. They're all there. Go and check if you don't believe me.'

I slipped through to the kitchen and came back with a few bottles. The issue dates and quantities left in the bottles tallied.

'These are all you have in the house?' I asked.

'What is this? Twenty bloody questions?'

'It's just that we have to be sure,' Paul said.

The phone rang and she picked it up before we got any further.

'Oh, it's you . . . Yes, I'm OK . . . No thanks to that wife of yours, she'd see me in hell given half a chance . . . It's the truth . . . Why have you sent an ambulance? No, I didn't!' She held the receiver out to Paul. 'It's Neil, he wants to speak to you.'

As Paul took the phone the doorbell sounded and I went to answer it. It was the two police officers sent to 'sort things out'. Before taking them into the living room I brought them up to date and said we didn't think she had taken an overdose. A couple of bottles of wine, yes, but no evidence of an overdose. Paul was still on the phone when I brought them through. The woman looked up, startled.

'What's this? I don't need the police!'

'Now don't get upset,' said one of the officers. 'We're only here to help. What's all this about an overdose?'

'Mary mother of Jesus.' She fixed him with a stare. 'For the last time, I haven't taken an overdose!'

Paul stuck a finger in his free ear and tried to continue his conversation with the son. Cupping his hand over the mouthpiece, he broke off and spoke to one of the policemen.

'Her son's convinced she's taken an overdose and wants to come round. Trouble is he lives a mile away and can't drive because he's had a drink, and as it's New Year's Eve he can't get hold of a taxi. He wants to know if you can go round and pick him up.'

The policeman looked at Paul. 'Tell me he's having a laugh.'

'The thing is,' I said, 'we can't leave her on her own threatening to take an overdose. She needs someone to be with her.'

The policeman thought about it, then, mumbling

something about not being a bloody taxi, went out to his car.

While we waited, the woman rambled on about her wretched life and how her hateful daughter-in-law blighted what little there was left of it. Nobody wanted her, nobody cared about her, and she might as well take an overdose. She was in the midst of telling us to make sure we didn't end up lonely and neglected like her in our old age when the policeman returned with her son. He was in his early thirties and looked as if he'd just been pulled from bed. His mother eyed him scornfully.

'So, it took a policeman to drag you round, did it?'

'Look, Mum, I don't want an argument. Why don't you just go to hospital in the ambulance? It's not fair you taking up their time like this.'

'You called them!'

'I know I did. You told me you'd taken an overdose, for God's sake!'

'No, I didn't . . . I said I was going to take one. There is a difference.'

'It doesn't matter, just get your coat.'

'I am not going to hospital. That wife of yours has brainwashed you, hasn't she? The evil bitch stops me seeing my own grandchildren, bans me from the house, and as for you! She treats you like a doormat and you just roll over and take it! You're spineless!'

Neil looked at us in embarrassment. 'She's had a bit of a drink. She always gets strung up after a few glasses of wine.'

'I am not drunk! But who would blame me if I was! That woman you married is the Antichrist . . . and you . . . you are her disciple! Those kids of yours are the only reason I don't end it all here and now. When I think of those poor little mites being brought up by her, well, it makes my heart weep.'

I was starting to take the view that bringing Neil round might not have been such a good idea after all, but I forced myself to look at the positive aspect – now he was here, we could all push off and leave them to it. Paul agreed it was time to go and as we edged towards the door the phone rang again. For the life of me I can't explain why, but I picked it up.

'Hello, Mrs Spencer's house.'

'Hello, who's that?' The voice was tentative.

'It's the ambulance service.'

'Ah, good. I'm Mike, Mrs Spencer's son. How is she?'

'Oh, er, not too bad, a bit emotional perhaps. Do you want to speak to her?'

'No!' he said quickly. 'I mean it might not be a good idea. We've had a bit of a falling out. Neil phoned me, I just wanted to check she was OK.'

'Neil's here. Shall I put him on?'

'No! We're not on very good terms at the moment. You know how it is, families and all that . . .'

His mother interrupted us. 'Is that Michael? Because if it is you can tell him I'm still alive . . . just in case he was hoping to see the back of me and sell the house.'

Oh God, we were off again. Michael overheard his mother's remarks and gave an unconvincing little chuckle.

'She always did have a bit of a sharp tongue on her. Anyway, if she's OK I'll let you get on, goodbye.'

He hung up before I could say anything else. His mother wasn't finished though, and we had to listen as we backed towards the door.

'He's another waste of space! New Year's Eve and he only phones to check I'm not dead. Do you know he moved to the south coast just to get away from me? Can you believe that? [Frankly, I could.] Doesn't even invite me for Christmas! What kind of son is that? [A sensible one, I would have said.] And what am I left with?' She looked at Neil and shook her head. 'I'm left with a son married to the daughter of Beelzebub!'

4.30 a.m.

Back in the ambulance Paul started on his paperwork while I considered my lot. It was half past four in the morning and I'd had just about enough. I was tired, hungry, thirsty and, more pressingly, I needed the toilet. Judging by the constant radio traffic all the other crews in the city were in the same boat, not that the knowledge made me feel any better. Paul filed his latest bit of handiwork and within seconds of booking available we were on our way to a man who had suffered a head injury. We were going to a neighbourhood unlikely ever to feature in *Homes and Gardens*. The area is dominated by brooding blocks of four-storey flats that wouldn't look out of place in a mining town in the Arctic Circle. Crumbling concrete, long windswept communal balconies, only one light in every four working, stray dogs rooting around the rubbish chutes – you get the picture.

Paul pushed tentatively at the metal security door and found that it swung open. If the dents and gouges over its surface were anything to go by, its 'security' status had been downgraded years before by the judicial use of a sledgehammer. The surprise was that the dents were on the outside. Someone trying to break out was understandable, but who in their right mind would want to break in? There was no lighting on the inside and it took a few seconds before we could make out the concrete staircase disappearing into the darkness above. With nothing on the wall to indicate where the different numbered flats were located, we headed up the stairs and out on to one of the balconies, where we were met with a blast of rain-laden wind. The first two flats had lost their numbers but, as luck would have it, the third flat proved to be the one we were looking for. The door was even more battle-scarred than the one downstairs. There was evidence of old repairs round the lock and further down were the scars of many a good kicking.

A human scarecrow opened the door. He was in his early thirties and dressed in a ragbag assortment of clothes that could only have been filched from one of those bin-liners you see left outside charity shops. His long hair fell in greasy slabs on either side of a face that looked as vacant as any face could look. When he recognized us it broke into something resembling a grin.

'Hey! It's the main men! We've been waiting for you, come in.' He took a step backwards, and then another to regain his balance. 'Whoops! Naughty, naughty. Had a few drinks, have we?'

He simply reeked of alcohol.

'Was it you who called us?' Paul sounded tired.

'Yeah, but strictly speaking it wasn't so much for me, it was more for my mate Pete. He's in the kitchen.'

'What's wrong with him?'

'What's wrong with him? Got a fuckin' rocket in the face, that's all. You should've seen it! Fizz . . . Bang . . . Smack!'

For effect, he gave himself a blow on the forehead with the palm of his hand that almost took him off his feet. 'It was like he got hit by one of those Cruise missiles the Yanks chuck around.'

'We better have a look then.' Paul sounded even more tired.

'Yeah, come in. S'cuse the mess, haven't had time to clean round today.'

We stepped inside and a cursory glance suggested that he hadn't found time to 'clean round' for the last couple of years and, by the smell, he shared the flat with a family of polecats.

Pete was standing by the kitchen door at the end of the hall. The only thing distinguishing him from his friend was a huge bruise centred on his left cheek. His eye was almost closed by the swelling. Paul moved closer for a better look.

'Looks like Mike Tyson's given him a pisser, don't it?' said the scarecrow.

Paul ignored him and spoke to Pete. 'When did this happen?'

'About two hours ago.'

'It's taken you two hours to call us?'

'I didn't call you . . . he did.' He gestured towards the scarecrow. 'I didn't want no ambulance.'

'OK, but now we're here you might as well tell us what's happened,' Paul said.

'We was letting off fireworks when this rocket wouldn't go off. I went to check it out . . . and bang!'

'You stuck your head over a lit rocket?' It had been a long night and Paul had just about used up his reserves of patience. 'What the hell were you doing letting off fireworks in the middle of the night anyway?'

'Why not? New Year, innit.'

'What about the neighbours?'

Pete looked a little bemused by the question. After a bit of thought he managed to come up with a reply.

'Fuck 'em.'

Shaking his head, Paul began going through the head-injury checks, leaving me at the mercy of the scarecrow.

197

'You blokes are the salt of the earth, you know. Know what I mean? You're sound! What would we do without you?' He shoved his hand towards me. 'Put it there, mate.' It's often said, and with some justification, that drunkenness can mask underlying conditions such as diabetes, head injury or stroke. There is, however, one certainty that you won't read in any emergency-aid textbook: it's only the drunk who wants to shake your hand. I've never had a diabetic or a stroke victim offer me their hand, but goodness, am I sick of shaking hands with drunks. I must have shaken hands with thousands of them, and have developed a kind of royal shake involving only my fingertips. Reluctantly, I went through with the ritual while he warmed to his theme.

'You must see some shit. Car smashes, people jumping off roofs, stuff like that . . . Ever been to a plane crash?'

'Not one that springs to mind.'

He looked disappointed. 'Wankers, I bet you get called out to some right wankers wasting your time, don't you?'

Yes, I thought.

Meanwhile Paul had finished examining Pete. He had been incredibly lucky. One inch higher and the rocket would have hit him smack in the eye. As it was, his cheekbone had taken the blow. Paul advised him to have it X-rayed as it might be fractured. His eye seemed to have escaped injury, but it was best to have it checked out. Pete didn't see it that way and, holding out his hand to be shaken, said, 'Thanks for coming. You're sound, but I'm not going to no hospital. How would I get back?'

Paul let go of his hand. 'Bus, taxi, you name it.'

'What, with no money?'

Funny how, when it came to money for beer and fireworks, there hadn't been a problem.

'Well, it's up to you. All I can do is advise you to come with us.' Paul picked up his bag ready to go.

'Hang on a minute! Hang on . . . just one minute . . .' The scarecrow, who'd been lounging against the wall, pushed himself free, only to stagger two steps across the hall and collide with the wall opposite. 'Oops, who put that there?' He looked round to see if we appreciated the wit but was met by two stony faces. 'Pete! You're going to hospital! These blokes didn't come here to be bollocked around.'

Pete, holding the doorframe for support, leaned forward at an impossible angle and came nose to nose with his friend.

'Read my fuckin' lips. I ain't going . . . no fuckin' . . . where!'

'We'll be off then,' Paul said as he turned to the door.

The scarecrow raised his palm in what he clearly intended to be a commanding manner.

'Hold on, stay where you are . . . he's going to hospital.'

'Sorry,' Paul snapped back, 'there's no point us hanging around if he doesn't want to go.'

'It's your job to make him go! You can't just bleedin' walk out.'

'Can't we? Just watch.'

5.10 a.m.

Back in the ambulance, it was a heavy-shouldered Paul who tore off a fresh report form and stared dreamily at the myriad of tick boxes. For a moment my conscience was pricked to the point where I actually considered offering to change seats with him. Instead, I opened my sandwich box, took out the German sausage and, before reason could overcome hunger, bit off a mouthful. Texturally, I don't think I would be doing it an injustice by saying it was like chewing on a condom stuffed with diced cattle tendons and tree bark. The herbs and spices in it, rather than enlivening the experience, rendered it all the worse by tasting musty and cloying. The one exception was the garlic. It came over strongly and as I chewed I began idly wondering what the atmosphere must have been like on board a U-boat two hundred feet beneath the North Atlantic. Not that I had long to dwell on the question. Paul had pressed the 'clear' button and earned us another job within seconds. Man assaulted. For goodness' sake, surely it wasn't unreasonable to expect that people would have got tired of hitting each other by now and gone to bed?

A downstairs light was on at the address and Paul, clutching the first aid bag to his chest as if it were a hot-water bottle, pressed the doorbell. A young woman came to the door. She was pretty even in her dressing gown and, above all, sober. My first thought was that we were at the wrong address.

'Ambulance?' Paul said.

She looked puzzled. 'I haven't called for an ambulance. You must have the wrong address.'

'Oh, I'm sorry. We were told someone had been assaulted here,' Paul said.

'No, sorry.'

'No, no. I'm sorry to have bothered you. Someone's got it wrong somewhere.'

'Not to worry, good night.' She smiled and closed the door.

We trudged back to the ambulance, where Paul filled in another report form.

'That's it. I'm not doing anything else until I've been to the toilet.'

I agreed. We hadn't been near a hospital for hours and all the coffee we had taken on board earlier wanted out. Paul picked up the radio mike and told Control about the last case and that we needed access to a toilet . . . as a matter of urgency. There was a pause.

'We have a 999. You're the only vehicle available.'

Paul was uncompromising. 'We need access to a toilet.'

This prompted a longer pause while the people in

Control presumably debated our human rights. In the end, the liberal faction won the day and we were directed to the nearest ambulance station, with the proviso that we hurry up. Feeling like a couple of schoolkids let out of the classroom, we headed off on the mile or so trip.

Halfway there I burped. It was only a tiny burp, a burp that would have gone unnoticed if it hadn't been for the overwhelming smell of garlic and mouldy herbs it produced. It took Paul two seconds to react.

'God! Can you smell that? One of us must have stood in dog crap. Check your shoes, will you?'

There was no point beating about the bush. 'It's not dog crap, it's my breath . . . Sorry.'

'Sorry! What the hell have you been eating?'

'It's that bloody sausage. It was all there was left.'

Paul threw me a menacing glance. 'Do it again and I swear I'll kill you. Justifiable homicide! That's the way the courts will see it . . . justifiable homicide.'

Ten minutes later we were ready to face the world again. Paul gave Control the good news and sat with pen poised. He wasn't kept waiting long.

'Do you still have details of the previous case? We've had the police back on the phone. They're adamant there's someone in the house needing hospital treatment. Will you return and check it out, please.'

Paul gripped the microphone and looked at me. 'They can't be serious. What am I supposed to say to the woman? "Oh hello, it's us again. Sorry about this, but we reckon you're lying. Can we come in and check round in case you haven't noticed someone bleeding to death on your living-room carpet?"' He was fuelling his own anger and before I could say anything he clicked the transmit button.

'Let me get this clear. When the woman tells us for a second time that she doesn't want an ambulance, what precisely do you expect me to say in reply?'

'We expect you to use your initiative.' There was an icy tolerance in the voice.

'This is a job for the police. Why aren't they going?' Paul said.

'We're speaking to them at the moment and trying to get some more information. Please proceed on the case.'

'Kiss my ass!' Paul hissed the words with such vehemence into the microphone that I snapped my head round in horror. His finger was well away from the 'transmit' button – it wasn't the first time he'd caught me like this.

'I tell you, Paul, one day you'll get it wrong and accidentally keep the button pressed, then there'll be hell to pay.'

There was nothing to be gained by both of us making fools of ourselves, so it was decided Paul should look a fool on his own. I stayed in the ambulance and watched as he made his way moodily down the path. When he was just about to press the bell Control came through on the radio again.

'Cancel your case. There's been a mistake.'

I gave a little beep on the horn and waved Paul back to the ambulance. Control was still talking as Paul got back in.

'The patient's not in the house . . .'

'You don't say,' Paul said to himself.

'There was a fight earlier in the evening and the police arrested somebody who now needs hospital treatment. The thing is, they gave us his home address when he's actually in custody at the local nick. We've sent another ambulance to pick him up. Stand by, we have details of another case for you.'

'So that's it?' Paul said. 'No "Sorry we didn't believe you," or even "Sorry you haven't had a break in the last seven hours"?'

I reached for my fruit trifle. I'd been saving it for last and, with my breath still reeking of Teutonic sausage, the sweet taste of fruit and cream would be more than welcome. I pulled off the lid and looked round for a spoon. There wasn't one. I had to overcome the sudden urge to chuck the thing at the windscreen.

6.00 a.m.

I looked down and listlessly watched the little green letters swim about the screen: 'Man with an arm injury in Aston.' He was waiting for us at the end of the street holding a blood-soaked dishtowel against his upper arm. I put him at about thirty-five years old, tall and well built with, I'm glad to say, an amiable smile on his face. He spoke first.

'Hello. I'm really, really sorry about calling you, I know you must be busy. Normally I wouldn't bother you, but I don't think this is going to sort itself out.'

He lifted the dishtowel from his arm and revealed a gaping wound in the large muscle of his shoulder. It was a clean cut that could only have been caused by a knife, or maybe glass. It was equally obvious that it was hours old. Paul took a closer look.

'How did this happen?'

'I was pissed, still am come to that. I think I fell and landed on a piece of piping sticking out the ground.'

This was rubbish, but Paul let it pass.

'Come on then, let's get you on the ambulance so I can have a better look.'

Once in the light we could see that a doctor was going to be kept busy with a needle and thread for quite some time. It was a deep cut and must have bled like the dickens, but by now a protective glaze of congealed blood had formed.

'Can you fix me up?'

'Fix you up? You must be joking. You need about a thousand stitches in that.' An exaggeration perhaps, but Paul was trying to make a point.

'A thousand! Do you really think so? I've never had stitches before; my body always looks after itself. Look.'

He turned his back and lifted his T-shirt, revealing

two ugly scars that had obviously healed on their own at some time in the past.

'Got them two years ago,' he said, lowering his T-shirt. 'Now, this one,' he raised his chin to show another ragged scar under the jawline, 'I picked up this one last year.'

'You should change the company you keep,' Paul said.

'You haven't seen anything yet!' He stood up and started to unbuckle his trouser belt. 'You've gotta see this little beauty to believe it . . .'

Paul looked aghast. 'OK, OK. We can't sit around admiring your—' He suddenly stopped talking and took a closer look at the injured arm. 'What's that purple ring round your elbow?'

'That's the mark the tourniquet left.'

'Tourniquet? Who put a tourniquet on you?'

'Nobody. I did it myself.'

Paul rubbed the grit from his eyes and sighed. 'OK, tell me from the beginning. What happened?'

'Well, like I said, I was pissed when I got cut. I went home and wrapped a towel round it, then I went to bed—'

Paul interrupted. 'How long ago was this?'

'Oh, I dunno. Two, maybe three hours ago. Anyway, the bed filled up with blood in no time, so I came up with the idea of the tourniquet.'

'Did it work?'

'Don't know. I fell asleep.'

'Well, I'll tell you something for nothing . . . it didn't! Tourniquets tend to work best when they're above the wound, not below it.'

'Oh, right, I see what you mean. That was a bit stupid of me.'

'No,' Paul spoke slowly, 'it wasn't a bit stupid . . . It was incredibly, unbelievably, mind-bogglingly stupid! If you hadn't woken up and taken it off you'd have lost your arm.'

If the bloke was offended by Paul's blunt assessment he didn't show it.

'Oh, right, I get your drift.'

'How does your arm feel now?'

'Bit numb. My fingers are stiff but I can still move them. No harm done.'

I looked at Paul. 'Shall we go?'

'Yes, the sooner the better as far as I'm concerned.'

We left the patient listening contritely as the triage nurse delivered a blistering lecture on the dangers of tourniquets and headed for the coffee machine. It was empty. We stared at it for a few seconds before Paul broke the silence.

'Let's go home.'

'There's ten minutes left of the shift – they could give us another job.'

'I don't care, I'll risk it if you will. I just want to go home.'

On the way back to the Street we spotted the drunk we'd plucked off the pavement earlier, head down as he doggedly weaved his way home against the driving rain.

'Do you realize,' Paul said, 'out of the whole night he was the only patient who really needed an ambulance?'

'Yes.' I tried to stifle a yawn. 'And the irony is that he probably won't remember a thing about it when he wakes up later.'

'Makes it all worthwhile, doesn't it?'

'Absolutely.'

Chapter Thirteen

The top half of Rudolph the Red-Nosed Reindeer appeared at the Street some time in mid-January back in that first year. Despite missing his rear end, he measured a respectable three feet from nose to midriff and looked so undeniably cute, with his forelegs drawn up tight as if he were leaping a chimney pot, that he quickly became something of a mascot. I first encountered him one night when Mike and I attended a hopeless drunk who'd been ejected from a pub and promptly fallen flat on his face.

Mike stood over the prone body with his hands on his hips.

'Billy! I might have known it would be you.'

'You've met him before then, Mike,' I said as we helped the bedraggled man to his feet and inspected his bleeding nose.

'Oh yes. We know each other well, don't we, Billy?'

'We do that, sir. All the ambulance people know me,

and they all say I'm the politest alcoholic they've ever met.' He looked round at me. 'What do you think, sir? Am I the politest alcoholic you've ever met?'

I looked at him askance. 'Er, yes, you probably are. Shall we get you on the ambulance?'

'Oh no, thank you, sir. Thank you for offering, but I don't want to go to hospital. If you could drop me off at a chip shop, I'd be most obliged.'

Mike rolled his eyes. 'Are you going to buy us some chips if we do?'

'I would love to, sir . . . but no, sir. No money, sir.'

Mike was smiling. 'If that's the case, it's no deal. You'll have to get there under your own steam.'

'Very good, sir. Thank you, sir.'

We let go of his arms and stepped back while he sorted out his balance. His face creased in concentration as he tried to remember how to get his legs moving. The message he eventually sent must have got jumbled somewhere en route as his legs suddenly, and simultaneously, set off in opposite directions. Startled, his upper body swung wildly back and forth in an effort to compensate before he somehow managed to swing one leg round to join the other. With forward momentum achieved by accident rather than design, he set off towards the road like a circus clown on stilts. Mike stepped forward and grabbed him as he neared the kerb.

'OK, that's it. You're going to get yourself run over if we leave you here.'

I opened the ambulance doors and helped Mike frogmarch the protesting man up the steps.

'Where are you taking me, sir?'

'Hospital,' Mike said.

'But I don't want to go to hospital, sir.'

'Yes, you do.'

'Honestly, sir, I don't.'

We heaved him into a seat and I clipped on the belt while Mike made a quick exit through the back doors and round to the driver's seat.

'Am I being polite to you, sir? Because I—' He broke off and stared at the stretcher. 'What's that?'

I looked round and saw Rudolph for the first time. He was tucked up under a blanket with his head comfortably on the pillow, regarding us fondly from big dreamy eyes. I stared at him in mystification, then turned back to Billy.

'What's what?'

'That!' He jabbed a finger at Rudolph.

I looked again. 'It's just a stretcher.'

'On the stretcher, sir! Under the blanket.'

'There's nothing under the blanket.'

Billy kept his eyes on the stubby antlers and bright red nose.

'Can you really not see it, sir? It's a beast of the forest with horns. Excuse my bad language, sir, but it looks like a bloody reindeer to me!'

'Sorry, Billy,' I said, 'but you must have overdone it tonight. Have you been on the gin?'

'No, sir! Just wine and vodka.'

'There you go then. Vodka's what they drink in Lapland.'

He gave me a pleading stare that nearly caused me a twang of guilt.

'I've been drinking vodka all my life, sir, and I've never seen a reindeer before. Honestly I haven't.'

I didn't know how or when Rudolph was slipped on to our stretcher. He could have been planted by a work-mate or, as we never locked the ambulances in those more innocent days, it might even have been a member of the public. When we arrived back at the Street I plonked Rudolph on the driver's seat of Larry's car and said nothing. From then on we vied with each other to leave him in the most unlikely places – in the fridge, the cooker, overhead cupboards, the boss's desk. He might even be sitting on the toilet seat waiting for you or hiding in the shower cubicle with a bar of soap on his head. Nowhere was off limits, and that included the ambulances. He must have travelled on scores of 999 cases, picking up as much experience as me in the process. Mike was always pleased to have him on board as it allowed him to tell me regularly, 'That bloody reindeer's more use than you!' – which wasn't fair because Rudolph spent most of his time in the linen cupboard.

He settled into the shift so well that one night Mike and I came back from a job to find our new friend propped up in a chair watching television while the others sat around discussing his name.

'H wants to call him Spot,' Larry said.

'Spot?' Mike asked.

'Yeah, Spot.' Larry smiled. 'Daft, isn't it? He hasn't a single bloody spot on him.'

'We've gone over this, and that's the whole point. If he did have spots, you wouldn't call him Spot. I mean . . .' H groped for some way of illustrating his point. 'You wouldn't dream of calling a Dalmatian Spot, would you, Mike?'

Mike seemed wrong-footed by the question. 'I don't know. I can't say it's ever crossed my mind.'

'Well, just for argument's sake . . . if you had a Dalmatian and called it Spot, it would sound stupid. Wouldn't it?'

'So you're saying that calling a reindeer Spot doesn't sound stupid?'

H was on the point of giving up. 'No . . . it's kind of ironic . . . Funny, if you like.'

'He's not white, so why don't we call him Snowy?' Steve chipped in.

Mike had heard enough. 'If it means I don't have to listen to any more of this rubbish, call the damned thing Spot and be done with it.' He cast me a glance and used a warmer tone. 'Fancy a cup of tea, Les?'

'Well, yes,' I said, not a little surprised. 'That would be nice.'

'That's good.' He slumped into a chair and picked up the paper. 'So do I.'

As winter tightened its grip, hot-water bottles took on the unlikely role of front-line equipment. Despite roaring away resolutely, the heaters in the Bedford ambulances rarely raised the temperature much, forcing us into overcoats and Spot into an old Aston Villa scarf. And if we felt uncomfortable as the thermometer dropped, then pity the poor patients. It can't be much fun being plucked from a cosy bed at 3 a.m. and taken out into a north-easterly. The elderly suffered more than most, falling victim to a plethora of seasonal dangers ranging from chest infections to slipping in the street. Chronic ailments, manageable in more clement weather, became problematic. There wasn't a great deal we could do for these underlying conditions but when it came to care and sympathy, we could deliver. It was an eye-opener to watch Mike, who ten minutes earlier might have been trading insults with a drunk, gently slip a hot-water bottle into an old lady's arms before engulfing her in blankets pre-warmed over a gas fire.

And it wasn't just the elderly who needed the occasional hot-water bottle. One freezing night in February two policemen spotted a young man weaving his way home along a canal towpath. They watched his progress from the comfort of their car until he suddenly lurched sideways and pitched into the water. When they reached the bank he was completely disorientated by the cold and splashing about, howling like a banshee. And it *was* cold. Stars were sparkling icily against a pitch-black sky while frost crackled underfoot like breaking glass. Not that the crisp beauty of the night was uppermost in the patient's thoughts; he was blue and shaking so violently he could hardly utter a coherent word when we arrived. All we could do was strip off his clothes and bury him in blankets with a couple of hot-water bottles thrown in for good measure. I doubt he ever thanked them, but if the policemen hadn't fished him out so promptly it would have been his last walk along a towpath.

Wintry weather, aided to no small extent by alcohol, was the cause of the first road death I attended. The pedestrian, a man in his sixties, left his local at closing time and rather than risk slipping on the ice-bound pavement, chose to walk in the road well out from the gutter with his back to the traffic. The driver of the car was making his way home from another pub after having had one drink too many. They met halfway down Lodge Road. The pedestrian died, and the driver's life was blighted.

He was leaning against the bonnet of his car, head in hands, sobbing when we arrived. Several feet away in the road lay a bundle of clothing that had once been a man. The heartbreaking scene was all the worse because there was nothing Larry and I could do for either man. After draping a blanket over the body, we stood with our hands in our pockets disconsolately kicking at the rutted ice and waited for the police. They quickly breathalysed and then arrested the driver for failing the test by the smallest margin. We had the task of transporting the body to the local hospital for certification before heading to the mortuary.

It was the first violent death I'd dealt with and as we lifted the broken body on to the stretcher, my mind went back to that rural road in France the previous summer. The red shoes, the pointlessness of it, welled up in my thoughts until Larry disturbed the flow.

'Oh well. It could have been worse. At least he got to the pub.'

I was startled. 'What do you mean by that?'

'If it was me,' Larry said, 'and you gave me the choice, I'd sooner get bumped off on the way back from the pub than on the way to it.'

I looked at him for a second, and then smiled. 'Yeah, you're right. It would have been tragic if he'd missed his last pint.'

Gallows humour – seldom funny, but often essential. Anyone listening from the sidelines would be appalled, but I was coming to see it as a means of hanging on to some kind of emotional equilibrium. I'm no philosopher, and I doubt Larry would put himself in that category either, but what's happened has happened, and no amount of introspection or self-indulgent brooding is going to change anything. That said, there has to be a way of bringing down the curtain on someone else's tragedy, and perhaps neutralizing it is one way. It could even be that hiding Spot about the depot like a bunch of schoolkids had therapeutic value – a kind of safety valve against what's occasionally thrown our way. But, as I said, I'm no philosopher.

If it wasn't snowing that winter, it was raining. The municipal sports fields were turned into windswept bogs with football pitches on which multicoloured swarms of players ranged back and forth like flowers tossed in a storm. Closer inspection of these 'flowers' usually revealed them to be mud-splattered, over-weight men trying to snatch back an hour and a half of their youth. And the injured player always seemed to come to grief at the furthest point from the park entrance. The temptation to drive out on to the field had to be resisted, as the chance of becoming bogged down was too high. Instead, the ambulance was abandoned at the gates and we'd end up taking a circuitous route across the sodden grass laden down with equipment we probably wouldn't need.

I hadn't been in the job long enough to be quite so cynical, but it didn't stop me mimicking Larry's groan when it came over the radio that we were to attend an injured footballer. I went through to the back of the ambulance to sort out the splints while Larry drove. I'd checked everything at the start of the shift but un-beknown to me someone had spirited Spot into the overhead locker some time later. His huge eyes stared at me from the recess but they'd long since lost their ability to surprise. I wished him good morning as I pulled out the splint bag and then closed the door on him.

We arrived at the playing fields to find a young lad waiting to show the way. He set off at a jog past the clubhouse towards the playing area and, defying convention, pointed to the nearest pitch, where a knot of players were gathered round a figure lying in the goalmouth. There hadn't been any recent rain and as it was a clear, crisp morning Larry broke the rules by driving the ambulance behind the goals and parking just a few feet from the injured player. He grabbed the first aid bag and jumped out as an anxious-looking lad came round to my side of the vehicle.

'He's in a bad way, mate, you'd better hurry.'

It's the kind of thing you get used to hearing, but something about his manner made me uneasy. I couldn't put my finger on it: maybe I read fear rather than panic in the lad's face, I don't know. Whatever it was, it caused me to hurry and join Larry. He was bending over the patient, who was wearing a bright green and yellow goalkeeper's jersey, and lying very still on his side in the recovery position. Larry wasn't speaking to him; he was looking for a pulse at the wrist while leaning his face down close to the lad's. Almost immediately his body stiffened.

'He's not breathing!'

My throat tightened as I crouched down and watched Larry's fingers move to the player's neck in search of a carotid pulse.

'I can't find anything. You try.'

I double-checked, but knew Larry wouldn't have missed a pulse if there were one to be found. Quickly and carefully, we rolled the lad on to his back. What had happened? Had he swallowed his tongue? A quick check. No, all was as it should be. Anything lodged in his throat, chewing gum or something? No, it was clear. This was crazy. With cardiac monitors and de-fibrillation machines still years away, Larry slipped an airway into the player's mouth before clamping the bag and mask over his face. He then began pumping air into him while I started cardiac compressions. As we fell into an automatic rhythm I could hear birdsong rising above the distant rumble of city traffic. From the pitches nearby came incoherent shouts and cries of players oblivious to the catastrophe unfolding close by.

As we worked, Larry tried to build a picture of events before the boy collapsed by tersely questioning the players standing round. The full enormity of what was happening in front of them was just starting to register, leaving them confused and frightened, but from the barrage of replies we were able to put together a picture. A corner kick had been taken and the goalkeeper had jumped unchallenged to catch the ball successfully in mid-flight. Clutching it to his chest he returned to earth, landed on his feet, then rolled over and lay holding the ball but not moving. Thinking him to be unconscious, his teammates put him in the recovery position and then called an ambulance. There was nothing in this description to give us a clue why he should have stopped breathing.

We carried on our efforts with dogged determination, which slowly turned to desperation. He was no more than eighteen years old; we couldn't allow his life to end like this on a football pitch. But every time we stopped and checked for signs of life, there were none. While we were making one of these checks someone scored a goal on the pitch next to us and a big cheer went up, leaving me with a hopeless sense of unreality. It was time to make a move. We'd spent long enough and the hospital wasn't too far away. Larry, as the more experienced member of the crew, would have to manage as best he could in the back while I drove.

My memory of the drive to hospital remains a hopeless blur of traffic and sirens. The staff had been forewarned and crowded round as we transferred the limp body on to a trolley in the resuscitation room while simultaneously trying to give an account of all that had happened. The tension in the room was beyond my experience, but every member of the team knew their own role and set about working with grim efficiency. Our part was over and we moved towards the door, where we lingered a while and watched. A nurse was cutting through the lad's jersey while another tied off the intubation tube that had just been inserted by one of the doctors. As I looked at him lying there, legs splayed and arms dangling, it was almost incomprehensible that this lifeless body had, just half an hour earlier, been brimming with vitality.

We wheeled the stretcher back out to the ambulance, paying scant heed to the small Salvation Army band preparing to play. It was their normal practice on a Sunday to stop outside the Casualty entrance and perform three or four hymns. The irony of their opening hymn, 'Abide with Me', wasn't lost on us. It had been adopted by English football fans before the war and is still sung at every FA Cup Final. For me, it became a melancholy sound forever associated with the death of the young footballer.

Unwilling to book clear immediately, we went back into the hospital and hid away in the coffee room. There was no gallows humour as we sat out twenty silent minutes gathering our thoughts. When we finally emerged and made our way down the corridor it took us past the closed doors of the resuscitation room. I pulled the door ajar and looked in. The fight for the boy's life was over and his body now lay on the trolley covered by a white sheet. I quietly closed the door and caught up with Larry outside.

The rest of the team had arrived and were gathered near the door, seemingly unwilling to go in. Most just stood on their own while a few had their arms round each other. They were too shocked for conversation and the oppressive silence was broken only by the occasional mumbled word. Seeing so much misery on the faces of people so young was hard to take and no one noticed us as we crossed to the ambulance. Back on board I picked up the splints from where they'd been abandoned and returned them to the cupboard. Spot stared out at me. I smiled at him forlornly. As far as I can remember, I never saw him again.

Chapter Fourteen

I learned later that the young footballer's brain stem had somehow become detached from his spinal cord. Even though no power on earth could have saved him, I was still left with an irrational sense of failure. Larry didn't seem keen on talking about it with me and when the rest of the shift were told the story I was surprised at how quickly they moved the conversation along by relating disturbing tales of their own.

It was a sobering discussion. But rather than deepening my gloom, I found it strangely cathartic as I learned to appreciate the innate value of sharing painful experiences. Affirmation that everyone on the shift held similar and often worse memories carried a significance that's difficult to measure. It was as if I were now part of a collective; a group of people who pooled their burdens rather than holding on to them in isolation. Could sharing memories dilute them and smooth out their jagged edges? Call it therapy if you will, whether accidental or not, there was no denying the value of these group discussions. I'd go as far as to say that twenty minutes spent talking with the shift is probably worth a hundred hours of a counsellor's time – not that counselling existed back then.

The mood on station never remained oppressive for long. It was too busy a place to allow that. The Street was the largest depot in the country at the time, with five or six front-line ambulances on the road at any given moment plus a host of 'clinic' vehicles operating between 8 a.m. and 6 p.m. Their function was to take patients to prearranged hospital appointments, and they were manned mainly by crews nearing retirement. From eight in the morning until early evening the place simply hummed with people and in the midst of the bustle was Phyllis the cook, our very own Welsh dragon.

Phyllis's function was to test our immune systems to destruction by serving food from a kitchen that would give a modern-day hygiene inspector apoplexy. Her culinary ambitions were modest, not extending much further than bangers and mash, and even then the results were erratic. But woe betide anyone with the temerity to raise so much as an eyebrow at the burnt offering placed in front of them. She might have been as thin as a lath, and not a great deal more than five feet tall, but her verbal onslaughts would have made Gordon Ramsay gasp. And I mustn't forget her able helper, Ken, the depot odd-job man. Not anyone's idea of an intellectual giant, to be sure, but a lovely little man blessed with a heart of solid gold. Unfortunately, personal hygiene wasn't a major priority in his life. The closest he ever came to washing his hands before buttering the toast was to run them through his heavily Brylcreemed hair and dry them off on his thighs. It was nothing to see him take a break from sorting the dirty linen and, smoothing down his hair, wander off to give Phyllis a hand in the kitchen. What with the invisible clouds of germs and viruses surrounding some patients, it was a constant source of wonder that any of us lasted a week.

The snooker table was the hub of activity during the day. It fitted comfortably into the messroom and still left plenty of space for tables and chairs. Mike was undisputably the best player and had long since been banned from entering the many knockout competitions we held. But that didn't stop him challenging and beating the eventual winner. There was an active social club organizing nights out, an air rifle club and, strangely, an angling club which at the time was engaged in dredging a lake somewhere in the country. The most popular form of socializing, though, was conducted just round the corner at the Hen and Chickens or, more often than not, the Royal George, a small pub not fifty yards from the back gates. My memory of those nights is rather clouded, but I doubt we behaved any better than the boozers we moaned about so vehemently when at work.

As for the Street itself, well, I don't think the architect was looking to win any awards for innovation or elegance. Built when post-war austerity demanded utilitarian features and nothing else, it was characterless and frankly beyond redemption. That said, I felt I'd been given membership of an exclusive club where I could mingle with, and learn from, a truly extraordinary group of individuals. My prevailing memories of those early days are of banter, wit and humour mixed with hard-won wisdom and, if you chipped away at the surface, genuine compassion for others. It's people that make a place, not bricks and mortar, and when colleagues from other ambulance stations referred to Henrietta Street as a dump I would think, yes, I suppose it is, but it's a happy dump, and I'm proud to be a part of it.

Mind you, they were a tough lot at the Street and rarely took prisoners. To hold your own in a conversation you had to be able to think fast and, more importantly, know what you were talking about: two reasons why I kept my mouth shut and stuck to what I knew best . . . making the tea. I was still working my passage, of course, but as that first winter dragged on I began to feel more at ease both with life on station and out on the road. I also came to appreciate just how tight a bond there was among shift mates. We could squabble among ourselves, but never in front of others. The very idea of taking a problem even as far as the first line of management was complete anathema.

The same rule applied to the depot as a whole. Maybe it was this united front that outsiders found intimidating.

We were also closely associated with the inner city and the amount of druggies, drunks and violence it generated. There wasn't much to be done about this of course, but I rather suspect most of us felt that if we could deal with the seamier side of life alongside the genuinely demanding cases and still come out smiling, then maybe we were a little bit special after all. We were special enough for someone to have coined the expression 'the Henrietta Street attitude'. It was commonly used and I was quite flattered, seeing it as meaning stoic, committed, trustworthy and professional. So it came as quite a shock when a new recruit stationed at some sleepy hollow miles from anywhere told me that he'd been specifically warned against developing the Henrietta Street attitude. When I pressed him to explain further, it seemed management regarded us as truculent, fractious, complaining, insubordinate and, generally speaking, best kept at arm's length. Bloody cheek!

Hearing this kind of guff only strengthened my attachment to the Street and, what's more, it may well have been the Henrietta Street attitude that helped save the life of a child. The accident happened just a few weeks after the death of the young footballer and involved a single car on a miserable, rainswept night. The first ambulance to arrive at the scene immediately called for a second vehicle and Steve and I were duly dispatched to assist. It was only a mile or so from the station and as I squinted through a rain-smeared windscreen at the dancing blue lights in the distance my pulse, as usual, started racing.

As the police car positioned to block off the road pulled aside to let us pass, I got my first glimpse of the crashed car straddling the pavement with its bonnet crushed against the side of a pub. Shielding my eyes against the glare of vehicle headlights and arc lamps set up by the fire brigade, I could make out several people huddled at the front of the car. Close by were two fire engines, a couple more police cars and the other ambulance. Their lights fired randomly into the night in a cadence of vivid blue flashes that left the pub seemingly at the centre of an electrical storm. Wet windows and walls throbbed to the light and puddles on the road added to the visual chaos by reflecting the image back tenfold.

Leaving the ambulance was like stepping into a devil's funfair. The fire tender's diesel engines created an almighty racket and belched clouds of acrid blue smoke as they idled at high revs to power the lamps. The noxious fumes hung languidly in the damp air until disturbed into ghostly swirls by silhouetted figures moving through the beams of blinding white light cast by lamps and headlights. I'd never experienced anything like it, and the tension I already felt was increased by the assault on my senses. And if this deliberately orchestrated nightmare fed my anxiety, what must it have been like for the victims caught up in the accident?

A fire officer, sparkling bright blue as the raindrops running down his face worked in rhythm with the lights, detached himself from the group round the car and made his way towards us. He gestured to the pub and said something I couldn't hear. Cupping his hands round his mouth, he shouted into my ear.

'Your patient is in the pub.'

As we were the second ambulance on the scene, I was obliged to report to the first crew and get their assessment of patient priority. I remembered that much from training school, and looked questioningly at Steve.

'I'll check the one in the pub,' he shouted back. 'You go and speak to the other crew and see what else they need.'

As I got closer to the car I could make out the woman driver still in her seat. She seemed to be conscious and trying to cooperate with the ambulance man helping her. The car's windscreen was shattered and her left arm stretched out on to the bonnet at a strange angle so that her head was drawn up close to the steering wheel. The other crew member was crouching in the front passenger seat shining his torch into the footwell, while a couple of firemen heaved at the driver's door in an attempt to get it open. As I walked round the car to join them I noticed three people, an adult and two children, sitting in the back. They appeared unharmed, but it seemed odd they should be left sitting alone in the dark while everyone's attention was focused on the driver.

I went round to my colleague at the front of the car and made my presence known by shouting over the noise. He was preoccupied with his patient but still managed to show his irritation by not looking up and shouting back curtly that he'd already told the fireman to direct us to the child in the pub.

'What about those three in the back of the car?' I asked.

Even above the racket of the fire engines there was no mistaking the dismissive tone in his voice.

'They're OK. It's the kid in the pub I don't like the look of. Just get him off to hospital, will you!'

I didn't recognize him and had no idea which depot he was from, but I didn't care much for his attitude even if the situation was stressful.

I made my way to the pub and found the injured boy sitting on a bar stool while Steve put the finishing touches to a bandage on his head.

'How is he?' I asked.

'You're fine, aren't you, Tiger?' He looked down at the lad and was rewarded with a shy smile. 'He's got a cut on his forehead that's bled a fair bit. It looks a lot worse than it is.' The child was alert and taking a healthy interest in his surroundings, which is always a good sign.

'So how did he get in here?' I asked.

'It sounds as if a member of the public brought him in.' Steve looked at the child again. 'You were in the front seat, weren't you, Mark?'

'Yes. But I had my seat belt on, honest.'

'I know you did,' Steve said. 'That was very clever of you.'

Seat belts were not yet obligatory, and were hardly ever used.

As we walked to the ambulance I told Steve about the people still in the car. He was surprised.

'Well, that's daft. Go and fetch them. The least we can do is get them in the warm.'

When I got back to the car they'd managed to open the driver's door but seemed to be having problems disentangling the woman's legs from the foot pedals.

'Are you still here?' It was the other ambulance man. 'I thought I told you to take that lad to hospital!'

'We've checked him out and he's OK. There's plenty of room for these three.'

'This woman and the lad with the head injury are the ones to worry about,' he snapped back angrily. 'If I need a third ambulance, I'll call for it. Now, for the last time, take your patient to hospital now or you're going to hear more about it later.'

It took a moment for the implied threat to sink in. If it had come from a shift mate I'd probably have scuttled off with my tail between my legs. But it wasn't a shift mate, and my hackles rose. I looked at the three bemused faces in the back of the car and made up my mind.

'I'm going to take them with me. You can like it or lump it.'

I opened the back door and strained to make myself heard.

'How are you three doing?'

The man shouted back, 'We're fine, just a bit shook up.'

'Let's have you all out then and get you in the warm.' Avoiding eye contact with my colleague, I stepped back as they slipped out of the car, the man first followed by the children, who I guess were around seven and eight years old. The second child seemed to move a bit slower than the first and, unlike his friend, showed no interest in all the activity going on around him. He was bathed in unnatural light but I could see he looked waxy and drawn. Instinctively, I scooped him up and headed for the ambulance; there wasn't any point trying to speak to him until we had some relative quiet.

My concern increased as I laid him on the stretcher. He was languid, preferring to close his eyes than look around. Steve moved across and as he quickly checked the lad from head to toe his frown deepened. When asked if he had any pain or discomfort the lad shook his head without opening his eyes.

'He's a horrible colour and his pulse is going like the dickens,' Steve said. 'I can't see any injuries but there's something going on. It could be something internal. Didn't the other crew check him out?'

'Yes, at least they said they had. I assumed he was safe to move.'

Steve was on his way to the driver's seat.

'Lesson number one for you: never assume anything. All you can do now is get him on oxygen and then hold on tight. I'll alert the hospital we're on the way.'

As we began to move I checked the child again. His abdomen was taut and hard, but it would be in an eight-year-old. Was that a suggestion of a bruise on his side? Maybe it was, but maybe it wasn't. He didn't react when I gently pressed on his stomach but he was becoming increasingly vacant. The only way to get a reaction now was by tweaking his ear. I was frightened – something was badly wrong; it could only be a head injury or internal injuries. Both Steve and I had checked his head with minute care – there wasn't a bump or a mark on it. Sweat mingled with the raindrops on his face. His breathing was becoming quicker. I checked his abdomen again and yes, there wasn't any doubt about the faint smudge of purple appearing under his ribs.

The waiting nurses whisked the little boy from our care the moment we arrived and disappeared into the resuscitation room in a flurry of gowns. We had to wait until the following day to learn the full extent of his injuries. His liver had been ruptured, probably when he was thrown against the seat in front. The Casualty doctor estimated that the degree of internal bleeding meant that without immediate surgery he wouldn't have lasted much more than thirty minutes. Thankfully, the operation went well and he was on course for a full recovery. I was stunned. Then it struck me I'd helped save the boy's life. I might have played only a small part in the process, but it wasn't without significance. What if I'd driven off with my first patient and left what turned out to be the real casualty in the car as I'd been told? If he'd been forced to wait for a third ambulance, which hadn't even been dispatched, then his chances would have been very slim indeed.

My first reaction was to give myself a pat on the back. Then, the more I mulled it over, the more uncomfortable I began to feel. Just how close had I come to leaving the three of them in the back of the car? There'd been a point when I almost had; I would have been following procedure after all. What was it that made me persist and enter into an unpleasant exchange with a senior colleague? Was it intuition? Was it devotion to duty or was it the bloody-minded Henrietta Street attitude that led me to face down an overbearing colleague? I still don't know to this day.

There was no getting away from the fact that the first ambulance crew had made a serious error of judgement. I don't know why. Perhaps they'd been caught up in the drama created by the three emergency services themselves. If Steve and I had been first on the scene, would we have behaved the same way? My self-congratulatory thoughts evaporated. Everything had worked out in the end, but I couldn't stop thinking, what if . . .

It's worth mentioning that the injuries sustained by the woman driver were relatively minor when compared with our patient's. She had a broken arm and a head injury that was in no way life-threatening. The lad with the cut forehead was discharged after treatment.

Chapter Fifteen

Life was going well. Marie and I had taken out a mortgage on our first house and despite having cleared out the bank we were full of optimism for the future. Watching every penny and searching through cards in post office windows for second-hand furniture wasn't a chore, it was an adventure. The adventure spilled over into work in more ways than I could have imagined. Although I was still very much the new boy, I felt I was gradually developing as a person. I was becoming more self-confident, assertive even. I doubt the others noticed, but I could feel it, even if experiences out on the road had the habit of knocking me back every now and again. Not that I was allowed to dwell on anything for too long. My shift mates saw to that.

I'd been partnered with Steve for several weeks and had come to admire him to the point of being starstruck. He possessed the qualities I yearned for: authority, charm, poise and a coolness under pressure that had to be seen to be appreciated. As with so many of the others at the Street, there was no hiding his military background. In his late forties, tall, ramrod straight, handsome and always immaculately turned out, he left me feeling like a scruffy shadow. It's not that I didn't do my best, but my unruly long hair and skinny frame condemned me to looking like Worzel Gummidge's younger brother the moment I donned my uniform. Steve rarely passed comment on my appearance, but when he did it was usually accompanied with a sigh and a lament for the passing of National Service.

He wasn't really one for high jinks so I was surprised and secretly delighted when one morning he set fire to the newspaper I was reading. Anyone careless enough to block his view of the messroom by holding the paper too high was considered fair game for this sort of thing. So far I'd been left alone. Being left out of the general horseplay rankled. I felt it set me apart, so with the first whoosh of heat came the gratification of knowing I'd gained some kind of acceptance. Of course I feigned anger as I danced out the flames on the parquet flooring, but as I cursed and swore terrible revenge, deep down I felt I'd reached a milestone, albeit an incomprehensible one to anyone on the outside.

Part of shift life I always looked forward to, with the proviso that Mike was nowhere near the kitchen, was the Sunday night meal. The city nightclubs didn't open on Sundays and the subsequent peace and quiet gave us the best chance we had of sitting down and tucking into what was usually pretty good food. Howard's curries were the talk of the depot, and we treasured him as the lord of the manor might treasure his personal chef de cuisine. He did have his eccentric side, though. One night he disappeared into the linen cupboard and reappeared with a large white sheet, which he spread neatly over the table. Intrigued, we watched as he tuned the old valve radio to a soft music channel and set the volume down low, then switched off most of the lights. After contemplating the scene for a few moments he unpursed his lips and slipped back into the kitchen, only to return with a ladle of curry sauce which he sprinkled randomly over the cloth.

'I don't want to seem nosy,' Larry said, 'but have you gone completely bonkers?'

'Ambience, Larry – just adding a little ambience,' H said. And then, breaking into an accent intended to evoke the foothills of Kashmir but falling somewhere between Welsh and Liverpudlian, he turned to the room. 'If you'd like to take your seats, gentlemen, the restaurant is open.'

We fell in with the joke, and when Mike metamorphosed into a very convincing restaurant drunk demanding pints of lager and side plates of chips off the bone, we were all in stitches. It was a good curry, but difficult to eat as Mike kept up his act with the rest of us joining in when we could. Then things were brought to an abrupt halt by a sudden howl from Larry.

'What the fuck's this?!' He was holding his dripping spoon at arm's length. 'Please, tell me I'm dreaming or I'll be sick!'

We leaned forward to inspect his spoon. Floating in the mixture of onion and chicken was a bottom set of false teeth.

H spoke through a mouthful of food. 'I was wondering where they'd got to.'

Larry dropped the spoon into his bowl and, pushing himself away from the table, stared in horror at Howard.

'You dirty rotten bastard!' He was having trouble controlling his voice. 'They're not yours, are they?'

H nonchalantly scooped up another helping of curry. 'Of course not!' he said, tipping the spoonful into his mouth. 'I found them on the floor of the ambulance a few weeks ago. Come to think of it, it wasn't long after some bastard dropped a load of snooker balls on my head.'

Larry bolted for the door with his hand over his mouth.

'The trouble with you, Larry,' H shouted after him, 'is you can't take a joke any more.'

It turned out to be one of those nights when the phone stayed silent. Nights like that don't come along very often and, not wanting to look a gift horse in the mouth, we settled down to relax in our own chosen ways. Video cassette players didn't exist, and the four TV stations closed down round about midnight, except on a Friday and Saturday when a couple of them might show a Hammer horror film. There wasn't even local radio. The only station to play through the night was Radio Two, and there's only so much you can take of 'Sing Something Simple' with Cliff Adams and the Adams Singers.

This dearth of external entertainment left us with little choice but to make our own. Card schools were popular, as were snooker, Scrabble and reading. Mike, Steve and I settled for a few games of Scrabble before easing back in our chairs with books and newspapers for company. Conversation waxed and waned and as the time drifted past I found it increasingly difficult to keep the words on the page in focus. I've never been one for sleeping on the night shift, purely because I feel so wretched when I wake up. But I defy anyone sprawled out in a comfortable chair at five thirty in the morning to stay awake. With the best will in the world it simply can't be done, and I allowed the book to slip on to my lap with the dreamy intention of resting my eyes for five minutes. Ten seconds later, or so it seemed, the emergency phone screeched into life, jarring every part of my being as effectively as a stun grenade going off in my pocket.

My arms jerked into the air and my right leg kicked out across the coffee table, scattering cups and magazines in its wake. A surge of half-digested curry welled up in the back of my throat as I snatched the phone from its cradle and, holding it at arm's length, waited for the wall clock to come into focus. I'd been asleep for an hour. A cheery voice on the other end of the line wished me good morning and, without waiting for me to reciprocate, passed details of the job. I copied them down mechanically and after replacing the receiver stared at the case sheet, trying to summon up the energy to move.

On the other side of the room Steve shifted in his chair and let out a gargantuan yawn.

'Bloody typical. We've done bugger all the whole night and twenty minutes before we're due to finish, they give us a job. What have we got? And you'd better not tell me it's an overdose!'

I was tempted to invent some outrageous job just to see his reaction, but thought better of it.

'We're in luck, it's just a maternity case.'

'Thank God for that.' He spoke through another shuddering yawn and, picking up his coat, headed for the door. Even though I wasn't capable of looking on the bright side of anything, he was right – it could have been a lot worse. If we had to go out so close to our finishing time then this was the job I would have chosen. What could be simpler than transporting a woman in labour to hospital? All we had to do was collect her, pop her in the ambulance and whisk her off to the maternity department. It wouldn't involve any physical effort and precious little in the way of mental effort.

There isn't much to be said for working through the

night, but driving on empty roads is a joy. It took less than five minutes to reach the address, putting us two minutes ahead of the schedule I'd been carefully mapping out in my head since we left station. If we spent a further three minutes getting the woman on board, then a five-minute drive to hospital, add, say, three minutes to drop her off, tag on what should be no more than a five-minute dash back to base, and bingo ... we would only be two minutes late finishing our shift. Such were the strange workings of a mind that given its own way would have keeled over and surrendered hours earlier. Not that I found anything strange about it at the time, quite the opposite in fact, and I was still fine-tuning my self-imposed timetable when we arrived at the address. Steve went to open the ambulance doors while I made my way to the house.

As soon as the door opened my little world, along with all my careful calculations, dissolved around me. One glance at the heavily pregnant Asian woman looming in the doorway was enough. She was standing awkwardly and breathing heavily, but what really alarmed me were those pursed lips. The way she stared distractedly over my shoulder into the middle distance didn't help either. I'd seen that preoccupied look before and knew it spelled trouble. Tentatively, I tried a greeting.

'Hello.'

Not much of a word really, but it had quite an effect. She threw both arms in the air, gave a piercing shriek and, while I remained rooted to the spot, toppled backwards like a felled tree.

It was only as I watched her fall that I noticed the group of adults and children crowding behind her. She was a stout woman and must have been quite a weight, but they stood their ground, catching her safely in a sea of hands before carefully lowering her to the floor, where she lay rolling her head from side to side chuntering to herself. I hadn't moved. It was not that I didn't want to; it was more a case of being unable to. I was transfixed. Part of my sluggish brain knew exactly what was going on, but the majority of it was in denial. Please, I was thinking, don't let this be happening, don't let her have a baby, not here, not now. All we need is another ten minutes. What's ten minutes as a percentage of nine months, for goodness' sake?

A teenage girl from the entourage crouched down behind the stricken woman and began vigorously fanning her with the hem of her sari while looking up at me in expectation. The entrance was narrow and the front door wouldn't open fully, making it difficult for me to worm my way in and squat down by the woman's feet. When I took stock, I found myself with my back jammed against the half-open door and my knees pressing into my chest. The woman was taking up all the space in front of me, her upper body lying across the threshold of the inner door and her shoulders almost touching the frame on either side. While I struggled, she dispelled any lingering hopes I had that this was all a bad dream by pulling her clothing up past her hips. Forget measuring cervixes and all that stuff: when a woman does that, she's about to deliver and no mistake.

My cramped position gave me little room for manoeuvre, but I did manage to bring one knee down on to the floor. This helped my balance, but the timing was unfortunate. At the moment my knee touched the tiles her legs parted and her waters broke. I tried to jerk myself upright but only succeeded in catching the edge of the door with my back so that it slammed shut violently behind me. This admittedly gave me a few extra inches, but with most of my weight now on one knee all I could do was watch as the fluid gushed around my shoes and soaked into my trousers.

Fighting back a string of expletives, I looked up at the family watching interestedly from the inner doorway. There were two men, three women, and several children about thigh height. Each clung to the nearest pair of adult legs as they jostled for the best view. When they saw me looking in their direction they froze open-mouthed, their impossibly large brown eyes set wide in angelic faces. I tried to give them a reassuring smile, but it must have been more of a tortured grimace as it succeeded only in making the smallest one burst into tears. A shifting of position from the woman brought me back to reality.

'Do you want to push?' The question froze on my lips as she let out a screech that in the confined space pierced me as effectively as a piece of shrapnel through the brain. It also triggered howls of anguish from the children. Howard's curry returned to the back of my throat as I looked down and found the woman was urinating.

I've read about people gaining superhuman strength in times of extreme adversity but, to my disappointment, I barely had the energy to move out of the way. I tried to heave myself into an upright position, only to be forced straight back down when I saw the baby's head appear. I cupped my hands close to the small portion of the wrinkled scalp visible and, as I waited for the next push, found time to feel sorry for myself. People aren't supposed to have babies lying on unforgiving tiles in cold, draughty hallways. They're supposed to be in bed engulfed in soft cotton sheets, jugs of hot water at the ready, blankets warming over an open fire, and with the comforting sight of an ample, rosy-cheeked midwife bustling about in the background.

The image was abruptly blotted out by her next push. The baby's head welled out into my hands, quickly followed by its shoulders. More often than not there's a pause before the next contraction, allowing time to check the position of the umbilical cord and generally get comfortable with the fact that everything's going as it should. But not this time. The baby's entrance into the world was achieved in one effortless push, leaving me flailing around trying to keep hold of him. For anyone who might one day have to catch a newborn baby, a word of warning: they're very slippery things. This one was no exception and I found myself juggling with him, terrified he might slip into the mess below. When I had him under control I looked down to make sure that the mother wasn't bleeding unduly. She wasn't, but fluid was still coming from her, adding substantially to the pool I was kneeling in. Not that I cared any more. My trousers had already soaked up as much as they could hold.

The important thing now was that the baby breathed in air and let out a healthy cry, which to my immense relief he did without any prompting from me. The children became animated behind the prostrate mother. Tears were forgotten as they jumped up and down clapping their hands and giggling into each other's faces – all except the little one, who still hadn't recovered from my reassuring smile and continued to wail. One of the men, his face lit up by the biggest grin I'd ever seen, said something to me in his own language while simultaneously giving me the thumbs-up. He must have been the father. I attempted to smile back at him but I doubt if it carried much conviction; from where I was kneeling there was precious little to smile about. I would have given anything for a swig of Gaviscon.

The persistent crying of the baby and the chattering laughter from the children echoing round the walls made the small space sound like Saturday morning at the local swimming baths. I was soaking wet, nauseous, and couldn't use my hands as they were clutching the baby. It wasn't possible to put him down because of the mess on the floor, and I couldn't lay him on the mother's abdomen as the amount of umbilical cord exposed wouldn't allow it. My back was still wedged against the door and I was unable to move forward. In short, I was trapped.

On the plus side, there was the baby. At least he wasn't a worry. He was a big, healthy-looking boy with plenty of energy. He had to be kept warm, but other than that he wasn't going to give me any trouble. What to do next was the real problem. I was working on it when Steve rang the doorbell. When he didn't get an immediate response he started banging on the door with all the subtlety of an early morning police raid. In front of me were the good-natured smiles and relieved chatter of the family, in my arms was a howling baby and below me a seemingly uninterested mother intent on going to sleep amid the din. I felt beleaguered and responded to Steve in a manner I normally wouldn't have dreamed of.

'Will you stop that bloody banging! Things are bad enough in here.'

I was rewarded by an offended silence and returned my attention to finding a way out of the mess. The obvious solution was for the two men to hook their arms under the woman's armpits and pull her backwards, then I could follow with the baby and Steve would be able to get through the door. It was a simple plan and the family listened carefully as I explained what I wanted them to do.

'OK, if you're ready,' I said, 'let's pull her back. One . . . two . . . three . . . pull.'

No one moved. It hadn't so much as crossed my mind that, on top of everything else, we might have a communications barrier. 'Does anyone speak English?' I put the question in hope rather than expectation. It drew sheepish looks before one of the heads nodded at me and said, 'Yes . . . no English.'

The knocking on the door behind me had started up again.

'Steve! Please stop banging. I'm holding a baby. I can't move. I can't open the door. I'm soaking wet, and nobody here speaks English.' There was a pause from the other side of the door while Steve considered the information. In fairness to him, all he'd seen was me entering the house and the door slamming shut a few seconds later.

'This is a joke . . . isn't it?'

It was all I needed. 'Can you hear me laughing?'

There was another pause.

'You're serious? She's actually had the baby?'

I gritted my teeth. 'Yes.'

'And you can't open the door?'

'No.'

'I can't take my eye off you for a minute, can I, Les? OK, I'll get on the radio for a midwife.'

I looked at the family. All it needed was for the woman to be pulled back into the house a foot or two. I tried to convey the idea by jerking my head vigorously towards the interior of the house while simultaneously flicking my eyes back and forth between the mother and them. I thought I'd made a pretty good job of getting the message across but, as their smiles were replaced by looks of genuine concern, I began to doubt it. If there was an initial adrenalin rush, and I'm not sure there had been, it was long gone, leaving me engulfed in a blanket of fatigue. My crouched position had restricted the circulation to my legs, so that one foot felt as if it were being attacked by a colony of soldier ants. When I'd just about given up, either as a result of my mime or of his own volition, the man with the grin took control. He gave instructions to the other man and together they started pulling the woman a few feet down the corridor while I hopped along behind, dragging my dead leg with me.

One of the women squeezed past and opened the front door, allowing Steve, armed with blankets, sheets and other paraphernalia, to step in. He looked at the mother on the floor, then at the baby, and finally at me.

'What on earth's been going on?'

'Oh Steve, please!' I handed him the baby. 'Here, take this.'

He looked at the child as if he were a ticking bomb while I straightened my back inch by inch and began hobbling about, furiously rubbing my legs in an attempt to get some circulation back into them. What was it I'd said to Steve when we were given the job? 'We're in luck; it's only a maternity case.' Not to tempt fate was a lesson I thought I'd learned, but obviously not.

Chapter Sixteen

The door opened just enough for the young man to scrutinize me through the gap. His face was contorted into an unpleasant grimace against the morning sunlight and, after holding my eye for a couple of seconds, he said, 'Hello?'

Slightly unnerved, I glanced questioningly at Larry, and then back at the unblinking eyes.

'Hello . . . you called for an ambulance?'

The question was considered carefully.

'Yes . . . I did.'

He seemed to be waiting for me to say something else and while I tried to figure out what it could be, Larry leaned over my shoulder and snapped impatiently, 'Well, we're here. Are you going to let us in or what?'

The eyes blinked for the first time.

'Yes, but you're too late.'

The door swung open and we got a proper look at him. Leaving aside the Hawaiian shirt, the first thing to strike me was his height. He couldn't have been more than eighteen but was well over six feet and already had a compensatory stoop. It didn't do anything to flatter a body so thin that it might have been a coat hanger under his shirt rather than a pair of shoulders. His wide-eyed stare was set in a gaunt, pasty face criss-crossed by patches of uneven stubble, suggesting he'd not only shaved in a hurry but also in the dark. The bizarre appearance was finished off by a wild mop of black hair perched on the top of his head like a heron's nest. I knew better than to look at Larry, but that didn't stop him whispering in my ear as we stepped inside, 'Christ, he looks like something out of *Carry on Screaming*.'

I turned my smile into what I hoped was a cheery greeting. 'Well then . . . how can we help you?'

His eyes flicked nervously about my face as he jutted his head forward.

'You've come too late . . . he's dead. I think he was dead before I got up.' The voice was high-pitched and, as he continued, went even higher. 'He's stiff and cold . . . he's had it!'

It was my turn to hesitate. There'd been nothing in the case as we were given it to suggest a sudden death.

'Who's dead?' I asked.

'My brother! Come and have a look, but I'm telling you, he's as dead as mutton.'

I might lack experience, but I'd never thought I'd hear someone describe a relative as being 'as dead as mutton'. But, as I reminded myself, people can behave strangely when they're in shock.

He led us into a dingy living room that by the looks of it had been exclusively furnished from a 1960s retro shop. It was reasonably clean but had a tired, worn-out feel to it. The flowered curtains were drawn, leaving a standard lamp crowned by a ghastly pink shade as the only source of illumination. Next to the lamp was a Formica coffee table piled with dirty mugs. On the other side of the room a black plastic settee faced the television. On the settee lay the unmistakable shape of a body covered by a blanket not quite big enough to hide it completely. The head was hidden, but a large pair of white feet lay exposed at the other end. The only sound was the solemn tick-tock of an old tin alarm clock on the mantelpiece.

I took a deep breath and crossed the room.

'Do you live here together?' I asked the question more to break the silence than anything else. Unfortunately, it hit a nerve in the young man and proved almost too much for him. He turned to face the wall in an effort to hide his grief.

'Yes, we've always been together . . . I thought we always would be . . . Oh God!'

The reply was choked off. Annoyed with myself for putting the question, I leaned over the body and pulled back the blanket. My glimpse of the corpse was brief. A pale face framed by black hair was all that registered before it exploded into life.

It jerked upright with an ear-piercing shriek, throwing its arms into the air high above my head. The opened hands fluttered for a brief second before the right one came down to its face. The thumb was swiftly placed on the nose, and the extended fingers were furiously waggled as the corpse blew a raspberry.

I reconstructed these movements in my mind later. At the time it was all a chaotic, heart-thumping blur, in the midst of which I heard myself let out the squeal of a piglet in distress. In the space of a heartbeat, and without knowing how, I was standing three feet from my original position staring at the apparition on the settee. The blanket had fallen back to its waist as it sat with rolling eyes and an inane grin.

I had only myself to blame. I'd known something wasn't quite right from the start and should have been on my guard; instead I became the dazed victim of a macabre practical joke. I looked round at the others, and then back at the 'corpse'. It was doubled up in a paroxysm of hysterical laughter; a second glance at its 'brother' showed him to be equally incapacitated. He was bent over, legs crossed at the knees, clutching his groin with one hand while beating the wall with the other. His face was a mixture of pain and ecstasy as he battled to avoid wetting himself. I wasn't expecting any moral support from Larry, so it didn't come as a surprise to see he'd joined in the laughter. His vantage point by the door not only separated him by a few feet from the raw shock of the Lazarus impersonation;

it also gave him the chance to savour my reaction.

When everyone eventually calmed down we got to the bottom of it all. It transpired that the two occupants of the house had until recently been residents in a local psychiatric hospital. The imminent closure of the hospital meant that these two, along with a lot of others, had been placed in a halfway house where they received their daily medication but were otherwise expected to fend for themselves.

It seemed they had developed, and perfected, their game of playing dead in the hospital, where it was repeated interminably. In terms of shock value, though, it must have become a game of diminishing returns and I can only imagine their delight on discovering themselves out in the world with a limitless supply of new and unwitting victims. It was just my bad luck that they chose an ambulance crew for a trial run. I tried to give them a stern lecture on wasting the service's time, and the general folly of their actions. They listened politely, nodding in agreement with everything I said, but I could see my words were falling on stony ground. The smiles never really left their faces, and the slightly detached look in their eyes spoke volumes. This game had only just started.

Larry was still laughing when we got back in the ambulance. I made a point of not looking at him.

'I don't see what's so bloody funny!'

'It was your face! I wish you could have seen your face! And that noise! You sounded like someone who'd dropped a lump hammer on his toe!' He pulled himself together and continued, 'For the life of me, I can't understand why you didn't smell a rat.'

'I did think something was—'

'The moment he opened the door I caught the whiff of a rat the size of a bloody elephant.' He started laughing again. 'I mean . . . the state of him! All he needed was Scooby Doo licking his face and it would have been perfect.'

'I was going to say—'

'And the Hawaiian shirt covered in fag burns! Surely that was a giveaway?'

'Fag burns?'

'Yeah. There's a dress code for these sort of people, and fag burns are an essential part. You'll soon come to recognize it.'

'Really.' I was looking out of the side window.

Larry sat smiling to himself. 'You know, when I pack in this job I'm going to open a shop. It'll be an exclusive outfitter for the gentleman loony about town. I'll have rows of brown corduroy trousers, all second-hand with the fly buttons missing, and all in one size: forty-six-inch waist, twenty-six-inch leg. There'll be racks of elasticated "S" belts and sets of red braces. Kipper ties with their ends cut off and Mexican sunsets printed on them. More pairs of white socks than you could shake a stick at. Brown brogues with run-down heels and different coloured laces.' He was on a roll and I couldn't have stopped him if I'd tried. 'And we mustn't forget the plimsolls and bumper boots. The biggest-selling line will be the multicoloured check shirts with their collar stiffeners poking through. And, last but not least, hideous jumpers that look like they've been made out of plasticine.'

At last he broke off and looked at me. 'What do you think?'

'I think you're nuts.'

'Don't be hasty, there might be a job in it for you. I'll need someone to sprinkle gravy and ketchup on the ties and jumpers before they go on display. And I'll need a doorman to make sure no one leaves the shop wearing anything that fits.'

'You've got it all figured out, haven't you,' I said.

'Yep, even the name. How does Larry's Loony Lingerie sound?'

Larry wasted no time in spreading the story of the 'corpse' to anyone who would listen back at the Street. Having been the butt of every conceivable joke about false teeth, he seized the chance to turn the spotlight on to someone else. Shift mates would jump out of doorways when they saw me coming, shout 'Boo!' and wave their arms about, then walk off laughing. Others whom I didn't know so well would just smile and shake their heads as we passed in the corridor, which was even worse. At one point Steve sat me down and asked what I'd been taught at training school about distinguishing the living from the dead. Even Phyllis was at it. She couldn't hand me a sausage sandwich without warning me to be careful it didn't jump off the plate at me.

Everything that goes round comes round, and it didn't take too long before I could turn the tables on Larry. We'd been called to a house where someone had collapsed with stomach pains. Larry was first up the path and as he reached out to ring the bell the door was violently flung open. Standing in front of us was a wild-eyed and very agitated woman.

'At last! Where have you been? Come on, he's in here!' Still talking, she led us across the hall to the living room. 'You simply have to take him away, I can't cope any more! How am I supposed to look after a sick man? It's not as if I'm well myself. The things I have to put up with! My doctor's very worried about me—'

She didn't pause for breath as Larry tried to get a word in. 'Where's—'

'He's had me up half the night fetching and carrying. I do my best but I'm only human, aren't I? At my age I should be taking things easy . . .'

Larry was the attendant that day so the onus was on him to take the lead and for me to assist when required. Two people asking questions can be confusing, so I stood back and watched with interest to see how he was going to deal with her. He drew himself up to his full height of six feet two, and in a loud voice spoke across her flow of words.

'Madam! Please! Calm down and show us where he is.'

At first it seemed to work. She stopped talking and looked at him quizzically. 'What do you mean?'

'I mean . . . where is he?' Larry repeated.

'Where is he? He's sitting right in front of you!' She pointed at an empty armchair.

Larry opened his mouth to speak but was obviously struggling to find the appropriate words. He looked at me. The case of the 'brothers' was still fresh in my memory and, with a warm feeling of expectation, I decided he was on his own. I avoided his gaze by ostentatiously studying my fingernails. Then the woman was off again.

'Don't take any nonsense from him. He never wants to go to hospital, but this time he simply has to go! My God, if you'd seen him in the night—'

Larry found his voice and broke in loudly. 'There's no one in the chair. Where is he?'

She stopped talking and gave him a long stare. 'Are you mad?' Before he could answer, she smiled knowingly. 'Oh, I see . . . yes, I see it all now. This is your way of getting out of taking him to hospital, isn't it? The last ambulance crew were no better. There are channels, you know, channels I can complain through, and don't think I don't know how to use them!'

As Larry spluttered I decided to check the rest of the house just in case there was anybody else home. There wasn't, and there was no evidence that she shared the house with anyone. I found a letter on the floor behind the front door and picked it up. It was addressed to a woman, which I assumed to be her. Next I flipped open the spring-loaded directory by the phone at D and jotted down the name and phone number of her doctor, then returned to the living room. Larry was gesturing towards the seat, his voice high-pitched in frustration.

'There's nobody here! Look!' And he sat down heavily in the chair. This demonstration had no effect; the woman's flow of words continued unabated. Larry closed his eyes as he prepared to ask the obvious question. 'Would you like to come to hospital with us?'

For an instant she looked startled, and then angry. She gave Larry another long stare.

'What? What did you say? You want to take me and leave a dying man! Is this the way the ambulance service behaves these days? Dear God!'

The only way I could think of extricating us was to call out her doctor and place the problem firmly in his lap. Leaving Larry being berated on his shortcomings, I strolled out to the ambulance and radioed Control. When I eventually got them to understand our predicament, I requested a doctor. They replied five minutes later that the doctor would be with us in half an hour and we were to stay with the patient until he arrived. Not much had changed when I got back to the room.

'. . . boiled sprouts, boiled cabbage and stewed prunes!' She was ticking the list off on her fingers. 'That's what his bowels need! If I've told him once I've told him a thousand times, but does he listen? No, of course he doesn't. Look after your bowels, I keep telling him, and your bowels will look after you . . .'

Larry was hunched in the chair. He'd given up trying to reason with her and simply let her voice wash over him. I gave him the news about the doctor and said I would wait in the ambulance until he arrived. Larry got to his feet, a look of alarm spreading over his face.

'You're not leaving me alone in here for half an hour!'

'Sorry, but yes. My place is by the radio.'

Our exchange went unnoticed by the woman, who droned on. 'Why don't you men ever listen to common sense? I could sort out his bowels at a stroke, but will he let me get at them? Oh no, of course he won't, they are his business, he says . . . his business! Ha! It's me that has to live with them! And then he has the nerve to complain about having difficult motions . . . I'll give him difficult motions!'

I closed the door on the way out.

The doctor arrived three quarters of an hour later, giving me plenty of time to read the paper and watch the world go by. It was a stony-faced Larry who eventually climbed into the ambulance and slammed the door shut.

'Well,' I said, 'did she sort out your bowels?'

He looked straight ahead and said, 'I'm not talking to you.'

Chapter Seventeen

I arrived at work to start the day shift in good spirits despite having scraped only about five hours' sleep. The early summer sun had risen an hour earlier and had already burned off any lingering traces of the dawn mist, leaving the sky blue and clear. It was going to be another lovely day and, come what may, I was going to enjoy it. When the last of the night shift trooped off home we settled into their chairs and what conversation there was confined itself to a gentle bickering about who should make the tea and toast. When it was finally agreed that it should be me, the only sounds to break the silence were the rustle of newspapers and the occasional muted snore. If there's a better way of starting the working day I'd like to hear about it.

When the emergency phone rang an hour later, a rejuvenated Larry answered it with an alacrity that must have startled the girl on the other end. A man had collapsed in a park about a mile away and within a couple of minutes Larry and I were bowling through the city in his direction. The sun was high up in a flawless sky, making it the kind of day that not only raised my spirits but also made me consider how lucky I was in my work. Unlike the people trapped in the surrounding office blocks, I had the open air, a sense of freedom and, most important of all, a totally unpredictable few hours in front of me.

As we negotiated the city traffic, cars pulled over, their drivers beckoning us past, only too happy to assist in a small way. Little children out with their mothers waved excitedly when they spotted us, and we smiled as we waved back. How many people going about their work are looked upon so fondly? Not many, I fancy, and I appreciated it.

We pulled up alongside an area of recently created open parkland made up of undulating grassy hillocks dotted with young trees. The overall effect was rather pleasing, or at least it would have been if it weren't marred by the sight of a scruffy middle-aged man spread out on the grass and dead to the world. I know it's wrong to prejudge situations, but even from several yards away it was obvious he was asleep, and if the couple of cider bottles lying at his side were anything to go by, he was drunk to boot. Determinedly clinging on to our optimistic mood, we wandered over and looked down into the grimy, bearded face. It was the picture of contentment. With eyes closed and arms folded neatly across his chest, he snored loudly and messily through a slack, gaping mouth.

Larry crouched down for a closer look, then glanced up at me.

'What did the poet say? . . . "A thing of beauty is a joy for ever"?' Returning his attention to the man, he spoke in a loud voice. 'Hello . . . hello there! Can you hear me?'

This didn't get any results, so he shouted a little louder, shaking the man by the shoulder. The beard twitched, the mouth closed with a smack, then one eye slowly opened. Larry made an effort to smile.

'Are you OK?'

For a couple of seconds the baleful eye scrutinized him, then he got his reply.

'Fuck off!'

Larry's head jerked backwards as though he'd been slapped in the face. It wasn't in response to being told to fuck off – something he was well used to – it was more to escape the stench of stale alcohol. Larry stared at the grass between his legs as if in deep contemplation, then looked up at me.

'Do you think he wants us to go?'

'No, Larry,' I said, 'it's the way you speak to people. I've told you before—'

I was interrupted by a booming voice loud enough to scatter the birds from the trees.

'Leave him alone, you bastards!'

Startled, we looked around. The voice seemed to come from somewhere to our right and, shading our eyes from the sun, we spotted a figure silhouetted on the crest of a hillock some thirty feet away. By the way he swayed as he tucked his shirt into his trousers, it looked as if he'd just staggered to his feet. Once satisfied with his appearance, he again yelled, 'Bastards!' and charged towards us. The charge wasn't very accomplished. He'd covered just five paces before the top half of his body was travelling faster than the bottom half – a situation that can have only one outcome. I watched with almost detached interest as he crashed to the ground and started to roll down the hill. His arms and legs flailed about as he attempted to slow his progress, but served only to propel him even faster. Like a log set free down a mountainside, he continued to gather pace. I would guess he weighed about fourteen stone, and with this added to his momentum he represented an unstoppable force. We were left with little choice but to step aside and watch as he headed towards the proverbial immovable object.

When we arrived, I'd parked the ambulance on the grass close to where the original man lay and, as luck would have it, this put it in the direct trajectory of the tumbling man. There was a dull thud as he struck the vehicle's wheel, then rolled back two feet and lay grunting in the grass. It's not often that we get the chance to witness our patients receiving their injuries and we'd watched fascinated.

'Well,' Larry said, 'that was pretty bloody impressive.'

'Wasn't it just!' I said.

Our would-be attacker seemed to be stunned rather than unconscious, and lay on his back mouthing incoherent obscenities at the sky. Nothing appeared to be broken, but there was a whacking bruise on the side of his head that left us with the tricky problem of what to do with him. He hadn't seemed very pleased to see us a few seconds earlier and there was no reason to believe his demeanour would improve any when he came round properly. He smelled like a pub carpet, but the effects of alcohol can be very similar to those of a head injury, and vice versa. This being the case, we were left with little choice but to treat his head injury seriously and take him to hospital. The sun was still shining, but not quite as brightly as before.

We unloaded the stretcher and lifted our newly created and, at this stage, uncomplaining patient on to it. In the meantime the original drunk had managed to get to his feet and now stood glaring at us. He was clenching and unclenching his fists, either to bring to the boil some inner fury or as a distraction while he searched for the words he eventually yelled at us.

'What the hell d'you two bastards think you're doing? Get your fucking hands off him!'

If you looked at things from his point of view I suppose he had a reasonable grievance. There he'd been, minding his own business and having a peaceful nap, when two strangers come along and rudely shake him awake. Not content with that, the strangers then knock out his friend and proceed to abduct him. He must have seen the whole episode as a conspiracy and was clearly winding himself up to attack us. Fortunately, he proved to be just as inept as his friend. When he took his first lunge towards us he found it necessary to take one step to the side, then two backwards to regain his balance, with the result that the harder he tried to get near us, the further away he got. Satisfied that he offered little in the way of a threat but still keeping a wary eye on his antics, we loaded his semi-conscious friend into the ambulance and I slammed the doors shut.

The drunk left outside had by now unintentionally executed a backward semicircle and found himself near the front of the vehicle, where he stood swaying from side to side and waiting for me. When I reached the driver's door he lurched forward with outstretched arms, displaying all the guile of an extra from a zombie film. I settled into the driver's seat and, resisting the temptation to run him over, started the engine and pulled slowly away. Behind me the patient on the stretcher was now fully awake and becoming increasingly irate; Larry was vainly trying to reason with him.

'Listen, you're in an ambulance! You've had a bang on the head and we're taking you to hospital.'

The reply was uncompromising. 'Like fuck you are! Undo these straps before I take 'em off myself and wrap 'em round your fuckin' neck!'

LES PRINGLE

'We're only trying to help you. Now lie back down before you fall off!'

'I'm telling you for the last time, you lanky streak of piss, let me off or you're going to get such a fuckin' smack!'

This was followed by muffled grunts and scuffling sounds. I eased off the accelerator and took a look in the interior mirror just as the drunk pushed roughly past Larry and made for the back doors. The ambulance was stationary now, and turning properly in my seat I watched Larry open the doors. The patient didn't wait for the step to be lowered and hit the ground running from a height of two feet. He managed a couple of wild strides before his legs got left behind for a second time and dumped him face down on the grass. The bearded zombie, who had somehow been trotting along behind us, sat down heavily beside his mate and draped a supporting arm round his shoulders. Larry stood for a moment to watch the pair and catch his breath, but when they started hurling fresh abuse and threats in his direction he slammed the doors shut. As we drove away I reflected on my earlier feelings of well-being and optimism, then gave a mental shrug. It was only eight thirty. The day would surely get better.

Larry still hadn't got it out of his system when we walked back into the messroom.

'If ever they invent an arm of medicine specializing in wankers, I'm going to be a bloody consultant!'

'I thought you were going to open a clothing shop for the feeble-minded,' I said.

'Forget that, there's more money in medicine. In fact, as I'm probably the country's leading authority, they'd have to give me a professorship. Lawrence Phillips, Professor in Wankerology. It's got a ring to it, hasn't it? I might even have my own column in the *Lancet*.'

'You might at that,' Steve said from behind his newspaper. 'As they say, it takes one to know one.'

'Now that's not fair, Steve. I can't help it if I'm on first-name terms with half the nutters and drunks in Birmingham. I'm sure they ask for me by name, and if I'm not on duty they call back later.'

The phone rang and Steve went to answer it. He wrote down a case and then handed the receiver to Larry.

'They've got a job for you as well. It's probably one of your mates wanting you to nip down the off-licence and pick up a few cans.'

Larry took the receiver with a sigh.

The case was passed as 'woman burned'. How badly, and under what circumstances, we would have to find out for ourselves. The lack of detail lulled us into thinking it was probably something of little consequence; perhaps a minor domestic incident like a scald or, as it was breakfast time, maybe an accident in the kitchen. It was nearly nine o'clock when Larry turned the ambulance into the quiet back street.

The sun was still shining and the scene was a picture of normality. A postman was pushing letters through the door of the adjoining house and the pavement was dotted with people going about their business and parents taking their bleary-eyed children to a junior school round the corner. But there was something about the elderly couple waiting for us on the doorstep that made me feel uneasy.

I couldn't put my finger on it; maybe it was the way they were standing. His arm round her shoulder, holding her close so no daylight came between them, while she leaned into him, the way a child might press against a parent for comfort rather than support. They were pale, displaying neither expectation nor relief on seeing us. They weren't beckoning; they weren't doing anything, just waiting. It was no more than a subliminal blink, but my unease mounted. Larry must have picked up the same message and didn't bother with a greeting when we reached them.

'What's happened?'

The woman looked up at Larry. 'It's awful, just awful . . .'

Her husband took over. 'Look, I think it's best if you go on through. She's in the back garden . . . she's dead.'

'Dead?' Larry stared at him. 'I don't understand. We were told that someone had been burned.'

The old man looked towards the house and in a flat voice said, 'She's been burned all right. Just go on through.'

There wasn't a hint of the acrid smell that even the smallest blaze leaves in the air. Everything in the street was normal too: no police cars, no fire engines, no fuss of any sort. Leaving the couple on the step, we made our way inside the house and immediately met a young woman partially blocking the hallway. She was trembling, and when I started to speak to her she just waved us towards the back of the house. The living-room door behind her was open and as we carried on through to the kitchen I caught sight of two small children sitting like statues on the settee. Everything in the kitchen was pretty much as it should be. Breakfast plates and cereal dishes were laid out neatly on the table; the only thing out of place was a chair pulled up in front of the sink and a pool of water on the floor nearby. The back door was open and we went out into the yard.

We weren't prepared for what we saw. Lying on the paving slabs a few feet from the door was a blackened corpse. It was charred to the point where it was hard to distinguish between melted clothes and flesh. One arm was drawn up with the hand doubled round, as if grasping for some invisible support. Shrunken eyes sunk deep into their orbits were directed upwards towards the blue sky. I took an involuntary step backwards and knocked into Larry. His sharp intake of breath came close to my ear and for a few seconds we said nothing as we tried to comprehend what we were looking at. Scattered all around were shreds of scorched clothing.

Fragments were also strewn across the small lawn and pieces hung from the bordering shrubs and plants as if marking out a grisly paperchase. It was Larry who broke the silence.

'How in the name of God has this happened?'

'I don't know,' I replied mechanically, unable to drag my eyes away from the body.

What I was looking at was so horrible, so incomprehensible, that it took time before my head cleared and I was able to look around for any signs of fire damage to the building or the garden. There was nothing. Other than the bits and pieces of blackened clothing and the corpse at our feet, nothing else had been affected. When we felt ready we went back inside. Larry carried on out to the ambulance to radio for the police and I looked round for the elderly couple. I found them in the back room sitting at the dining table, his hand clasped over hers. I pulled up a chair and joined them. The old man was preoccupied and I thought he hadn't noticed me until he dragged his eyes away from the tablecloth and looked across. Then, without any prompting, he began talking. After a faltering start he seemed anxious to describe what he'd seen.

They were next-door neighbours. Half an hour earlier they'd been enjoying the early morning sunshine while finishing breakfast on the veranda of their kitchen. He was reaching to pour himself a cup of tea when flames suddenly shot up above the wooden fence from the garden next door. His first thoughts were of annoyance that their neighbours had lit a bonfire on such a lovely morning. The flames had been so sudden, and so high, that he assumed the bonfire had been ignited with petrol, and was saying as much to his wife when the blaze began to move. He was confused; what he was seeing didn't make any sense. He and his wife followed the progress of the flames as they danced above the fence and travelled the length of the small garden. After a few seconds there was a single, sustained, high-pitched scream and, as it died away, he became aware of the hysterical squealing of children's voices. He got to his feet but could only stand transfixed as the flames moved faster and faster, then came to a sudden halt.

At last galvanized into action, he rushed out of the kitchen and ran as best he could down the communal alleyway between the two houses. The screaming had stopped by the time he entered his neighbour's garden and the first thing he saw, just a few feet from the gate, was what he thought to be a bundle of burning rags on the ground. A child was emptying a cup of water on to it, which hissed and spat as it made contact with the dying flames. He felt a sudden wave of relief at the thought that it was only childish mischief after all. It was as he reached forward to pull the child away that he saw it wasn't rags burning, but the body of a woman. With the child in his grasp he fell back against the wall of the house before stumbling into the kitchen, where he found another child on his toes at the sink filling a cup of water. He freely admitted that by now it had all become too much for him and, with the body still smouldering, he fled out into the street desperately looking for help.

The young woman we'd met in the hall a couple of minutes earlier happened to be passing and, seeing his distress, came over to see if she could do anything. All he could tell her was that there had been a terrible accident in the garden, and she should go inside and help the children. He then went back to his own house and dialled 999. Given the state he was now in, he could only get a few words out, which went some way to explain the scant details we'd received earlier. In the meantime, the woman had made her way through to the garden and found the children still pouring water on the body. She pulled them away and took them into the front room, where they stayed until we arrived ten minutes later.

When he finished I searched for something to say. But what is there to say to people who have witnessed a scene so horrific that it will live with them for ever? It was either silence or an exchange of banalities. How long had they been neighbours? What was she like? Was she married? We talked about anything that would distract our thoughts until Larry came back to say that the police were on the way and a doctor too, in the hope that he might be able to offer some kind of help to the elderly couple. Then there were the children to think about, two boys aged five and seven. Larry said the young woman was still sitting with them in the front room and, as two strangers in uniform, it was probably best we stayed well away from them.

Fifteen minutes later and the police had taken charge. A woman officer had been assigned to care for the children and a doctor was sitting with the couple in the back room. The Coroner's Office would take charge of the body, so there was no reason for us to stay any longer. On the way out we met the woman who'd been looking after the children. I stopped to thank her and asked if the youngsters had said anything. She sat on the stairs and went over the fragments of the story she had managed to glean.

The picture she put together started with normal early morning activity in the house. The children's mother had woken them as usual and supervised them as they dressed for school. Later, downstairs, she gave them breakfast. While they were eating she went out into the backyard, poured a can of petrol over herself and struck a match. The children did the only thing they could think of, which was to fill cups with water and chase their screaming mother round the garden, throwing the water at her while they screamed themselves.

Back in the ambulance, all I could see was a picture of the children chasing after their mother with cups of water. It went round and round in my head. I picked up the microphone to book clear, but then put it back in its cradle. What I couldn't understand was why it was an imaginary scene that lingered. I could banish what I'd actually seen to some recess of my mind, but I couldn't find anywhere to send the images I'd created for myself. Larry broke in on my thoughts.

'You might as well speak to Control before they start chasing us.'

He was right. Gloomily aware that it was only nine thirty and the bulk of the working day lay in front of us, I contacted Control and told them the police had taken over. There was a short pause before the controller responded.

'Further 999 for you . . .'

Chapter Eighteen

The others considered the grisly death of the young mother over our next shift meal. Larry sombrely ran through the sequence of events and in doing so managed to dampen the atmosphere round the table even more effectively than Mike's spicy Thai chicken. After a respectful silence Steve opened the batting with a story of his own.

'I went out to something similar myself. I think it was Buxton Road in Handsworth, where the council houses are in blocks of three. A woman went out on to the front doorstep and did the same thing. She went up like a torch apparently. When we got there a neighbour was putting her out with a fire extinguisher.' Steve took a nibble of chicken. 'The weird thing was that the very next night we were called to the house at the other end of the block of three. A two-year-old had been used as a punchbag by his stepfather.'

'How was he?' Larry asked.

'Died the next day. I've always wondered what the family living in the middle house made of it all.'

Howard tried to lighten up the proceedings. 'I got called to a man who'd climbed into one of those electricity sub-stations. He got fried big time. You could smell it from thirty—'

'That's enough!' Mike brought the palm of his hand down on the table. 'You're putting me off my food. Talk about something else, for Christ's sake!'

Silence. Larry was pushing a piece of chicken round his plate.

'So where did you pick up this recipe, Mike?'

'Malaya.'

'Oh, how long did you spend out there?'

'On and off, about four years. We were sent in to carry out raids across the border into Indonesia. Then I did a stint attached to the medical corps. The natives knew me as Lord Medicine.'

'What!' Larry was doing his best not to smile.

Mike cast him a warning look. 'Field Marshal Templer came up with the idea of ingratiating ourselves with the locals. I'm pretty sure it was him who coined the phrase "winning hearts and minds". Every village we visited on patrol was given free medical help. They loved us, especially when we lobbed the odd hand grenade into the river to stun the fish for them. The whole village would stand downstream waiting to scoop up the catch as it floated past.'

'So you gathered recipes as you went along?' Larry asked.

'More or less. The trouble is you can't get half the ingredients over here. The best thing I ever tasted was baked snake. You wrap it in palm leaves, place it on hot stones in a shallow pit, and then cover it with earth. An hour later it's melting in your mouth.'

Steve was never far behind when it came to recalling army days. 'Have you ever tried stewed puffin, Mike?'

Mike smiled. 'Can't say I have. Puffins were a bit thin on the ground out in the Far East.'

'Well, there's no shortage of them up in the Hebrides at breeding time. I was stationed there for a bit in the sixties when they were doing rocket tests. Rocks and sea birds, that's all there was.' Steve patted his pockets, searching for his pipe. 'The seagulls were pests. One in particular used to dive bomb us whenever we left the hut, so one day we got some carbide – remember carbide, Mike?'

'Of course I do. Nasty stuff.'

Steve noticed my puzzled expression. 'We used carbide in the lamps. It's inert until you wet it, then it gives off a highly flammable gas. So anyway, we got this lump of carbide, dipped it in water, wrapped it in bread and threw it up in the air when the gull was doing a sweep. He took it down in one gulp and a couple of seconds later came in for a crash landing . . . then he more or less blew up.'

'You cruel bastard!' H said. 'That was a disgraceful thing to do!'

'I suppose it was.' Steve lit his pipe and waved the match out. 'But this particular bird was a threat to life and limb. It was the size of a turkey, and came out of the sky at thirty miles an hour.'

'Anyway,' Mike said, 'you haven't told us what stewed puffin's like.'

'I've never tasted anything quite so vile in all my life.' Steve wafted away a cloud of smoke. 'I doubt you'll ever see it on a menu but, if you do, take my advice and give it a wide berth. It's like eating compressed seaweed and rotten sardines.'

For the next fifteen minutes everybody tried to outdo each other in describing all the outlandish meals they'd ever eaten. By the time Mike launched into an account of frying beetles in vinegar and black pepper on an upturned shovel in Swaziland during the 1964 asbestos mine riots, I'd all but forgotten the horrors of the little back garden. In fact, so immersed was I that I broke my own rule and joined in the conversation when the beetle saga drew to a close.

'If ever you want something tasty to wash a meal down with, Mike, I can recommend amniotic fluid.'

All heads turned in my direction.

'That's something you can vouch for, I presume?' Larry said from the other end of the table.

'Oh yes. I had a mouthful last week when I was working with Ron Smith from D shift.' To my amazement, I had the attention of the others for the first time.

Ron and I had called to collect a woman in labour and were surprised to be met by her sister and taken straight through to the kitchen. Our patient was lying across the breakfast table with her head resting on a pillow. She turned in my direction and, smiling, said, 'I want to push.'

Ron turned on his heel to go and fetch our maternity bag, leaving me to check the woman out. I felt uncomfortable, but there was no way round it.

'Is it OK if I have a look and see if anything's happening?' I asked, as I moved round the table.

'Of course you can, love.' She parted her legs a bit further. 'It's not a time to stand on ceremony.'

As she was at table height I only had to crouch slightly to get in line. Timing is everything in life, and on this occasion mine was perfect. At the exact moment I got into position, her waters broke.

You might imagine that, when a woman's waters break, the fluid oozes gently from her. It wasn't quite like that. It was as though someone had sucked water into a bicycle pump and then ejected it with all their strength. The horizontal jet struck me just above the heart and ricocheted off in all directions. It splashed up into my mouth, my nose, my eyes and my hair. The rest went down my shirt and quickly drained into my trousers.

I spluttered and coughed and, rubbing my eyes on

my shirt sleeve, raised my dripping head to look at the woman. She stared back in surprise and disbelief and started to apologize, over and over. I was trying to tell her it wasn't her fault when she began to laugh. I don't know if it was the emotion of the moment or embarrassment, but her laughter, mixed with apologies, continued until the next contraction.

'I only met you a minute ago,' she said, 'and I go and do that to you! I'm not a lady, am I? It's so embarrassing, and I'm so sorry.' Then she started laughing again.

The only good thing to come of it was that, as I needed a shower and a change of clothes, we could call for another ambulance to take over.

Some people can survive ten years in the ambulance service without being called on to deliver a single baby. I was excluded from joining that happy club very early on in my career. In fact, there were times when it seemed I only had to glance at a woman to send her into labour. And it's the strangest thing but I have no recollection of the first birth I attended. Short of visiting a hypnotherapist, I've done all I can to jog the memory free but to no avail. I can only put it down to having been involved with so many deliveries that it's just the more unusual ones that have stuck in my mind.

From that first eighteen months three are etched on my memory. I've already mentioned the woman who blocked the hallway; another experience was played out in the upstairs bedroom of a terraced house in Handsworth.

An elderly Asian woman in a voluminous sari that all but engulfed her tiny frame was waiting on the doorstep. Her bony hands knotted and unknotted as she gazed at us beseechingly and launched into an excited stream of Urdu. We'd come to collect a pregnant woman and, although we were unable to understand a single word she said, the old lady's message came across only too clearly: 'Thank God you're here! My granddaughter's having a baby, come quickly!'

With her eyes darting between us like fireflies, and still talking fast, the woman backed into the house and quickly turned towards the stairs. Larry and I exchanged a look of martyrs about to meet their fate.

'I'll go and get our stuff,' he said, and began to retrace his steps, leaving me to follow the woman up the narrow staircase. When we turned into a bedroom any lingering hope that I'd read things wrongly was snuffed out. The patient was leaning heavily against a chest of drawers, her legs wide apart and her features twisted into a grimace, as she battled with a long and painful contraction.

I waited for her face to relax a little before speaking. 'You OK? Has the contraction finished?'

She stared through me as if in a dream, then gave a long moan. Mingled with the look of pain, she had the tight mouth, the puffed cheeks and, most telling of all, that unmistakable air of total concentration. There was no doubt about it: even I could see she was pushing.

'You're not pushing, are you?' I was talking to

myself. I really wanted to say, don't push . . . whatever you do, don't push! Stubbornly, I stuck to the same tack. 'You're not bearing down, are you?'

She didn't reply and I waited for the second contraction to wane. Only then did she give me the briefest of mute glances and in it I read the answer to my next question.

'Do you speak English?'

She shook her head.

So there it was. Neither woman spoke English.

I coaxed her over to the bed, where she lay back against a mound of cushions. There are times when it's tempting to snatch the patient and make a run for the nearest hospital, but that wasn't an option in this case. It's not always so clear-cut. If we get it wrong and call for help prematurely, we're left trying to justify ourselves to a pretty frosty midwife. On the other hand, if our judgement proves to be over-optimistic the baby could be born in the ambulance, and that's by far the worst option.

Larry arrived, took in the scene and opened the maternity pack on to a nearby table to check its contents: gloves, plastic apron, sterile sheets, cord clamps, mucus extractor, sanitary towels, absorbent lint and scissors. (If I had anything to do with stocking these packs I'd be tempted to add a little handwritten note saying, 'Good luck.') Larry draped a couple of sheets over the radiator and went back downstairs to ask Control to send a midwife.

I donned the gloves and apron while deciding how to tackle the next step. I needed to remove the mother-to-be's lower clothing and get into position to see exactly what was going on. This would take some tact. Hoisting my bright green plastic apron up to my hips and nodding vigorously at her, I tried to mime that I wanted her to pull up her clothes. She watched me gravely and lifted her skirts without a qualm. With more urgent things to worry about, modesty was not an issue.

With everything now in place, I glanced up at her. She'd lost interest in me. Her eyes were closed, and the beginnings of another long wail slowly etched themselves across her face. My eyes darted back down just in time to see the top of the baby's head nudge into the world. So far so good . . . it might have been a foot.

When a birth is straightforward it's not me who 'delivers' the baby; it's the mother. I can assist by supporting the head and prevent it being shot into the world too violently. I can guide it away from the pool of body fluids that will have gathered. I can check the cord isn't wrapped round the neck, and that the baby's mouth and nose are free of mucus, but when all's said and done it's the mother who does the work. And as for witnessing the 'miracle of childbirth', believe me, you're too busy giving thanks that nothing's gone wrong to consider you might be participating in a miracle.

When it's over and the baby is in your arms, you

wait for it to take its first lungful of air. Only then can you start breathing again yourself. On this occasion, events moved so quickly I didn't have a chance to give thanks or hold my breath before I found myself clutching a healthy baby boy. His high-pitched cries drowned out my sigh of relief. The placenta was still inside the mother, leaving about eight inches of the umbilical cord exposed. My first priority was to get the baby wrapped up and warm. I was loath to lay him down because the sheets were wet and cold and the cord was too short to allow me to give him to his mother. The sheets warming over the radiator were out of reach and the patient's grandmother was standing quietly in a corner of the room. If I could get her to hold the baby it would leave me free to sort things out and get him wrapped up and settled on the mother's stomach where he would be snug and warm. Resorting to mime, I held the baby towards the old woman as if offering a sacrifice. She came near and I handed over my burden. This marked the point where an everyday delivery turned into something memorable, and for all the wrong reasons.

As I reached for the sheets I was suddenly aware out of the corner of my eye that the grandmother was walking away with the baby in her arms. I swung round in alarm, just in time to see the umbilical cord snap in the middle under the strain.

Umbilical cords are very tough, rubbery things and if somebody had told me that one could snap so easily

I wouldn't have believed them. We weren't allowed to cut and clamp the cord for fear of introducing infection, and as blood from the broken lifeline pulsed on to the bed sheets I lunged forward and grabbed the severed ends. Sweat broke out on my forehead and my knees felt weak at the thought of what damage might have been done. Fearfully, I leaned over to check that the mother wasn't bleeding after the sudden wrench on the placenta. Thank heaven, everything seemed to be OK. Then I checked the baby and to my relief he seemed none the worse. I let out a long breath. How could the grandmother have done such a stupid thing? Then it dawned on me that the poor woman probably hadn't been aware that the cord was still attached. What I'd taken to be obvious wasn't necessarily obvious to her. It was my fault.

I reviewed the situation grimly. The mother was lying on the bed with one half of the umbilical cord stretching up from her into my left hand. My right hand gripped the other end of the cord, which stretched to the baby still nestling in the grandmother's arms. I couldn't communicate with either woman other than by nods and gestures and Larry hadn't reappeared. Resisting panic, I eased as near to the window as I could and peered down at the ambulance. Larry was sitting in the cab chatting to some local kids who'd gathered round, as they often do when they spot an ambulance in their street. I stared at him, willing him to look up; but in vain. I shifted my gaze to the grandmother and she smiled back. I looked at the mother and, for the first time, she smiled. Both were confident that things were under control.

The baby's cries brought me back to reality. I had to get him covered up and warm. I eased the pressure on one end of the cord and when blood dribbled on to my hand I held it tight again. Using my head and the little arm movement I had, I gesticulated towards the sheets. The grandmother followed my gaze and, freeing one hand, reached across and plucked one of them from the radiator, then deftly wrapped up the baby. In the meantime the mother pulled some blankets over herself.

How had I got myself into this pickle? I felt ludicrous and inept; all I could do was periodically check the two patients, who were thankfully doing fine. The grandmother sat down on the end of the bed and I found a little space to sit between the two women. I'd decided to remain a human clamp until things could be done properly and sat clutching the ends of the cord while they chatted happily across me in Urdu. It seemed like an eternity, but it was probably only five minutes before the door opened and the midwife bustled in with Larry carrying her bag. I waited for one of them to say something while I stared at my feet.

'You four look very cosy.' It was the midwife's rich West Indian accent. Then she must have spotted the cord. 'What on earth's been going on?'

* * *

Not many weeks later I was again overcome by events. The patient had only been in the country a matter of weeks and didn't speak English. That in itself shouldn't have been a problem, especially as a neighbour was there to translate. She took us through to the living room where the pregnant lady was standing by the settee, looking decidedly ill at ease. She cast a furtive glance our way and then took a keen interest in her sleeve, steadfastly refusing to look in our direction again.

It could have been shyness, but more probably she was disconcerted to find that two men had been sent to look after her. Whatever the reason, she shifted her weight from foot to foot with head bowed as we tried to get some basic information via her neighbour. We didn't need to find out much: all we wanted to know was the length of time between the contractions and if her waters had broken. I asked the interpreter to put these two simple questions to the woman. After a fairly long exchange, the neighbour turned to me and said, 'She doesn't know.'

'She doesn't know what?'

'She doesn't know if her waters have broken or if she is having contractions.'

'She must know,' I said. 'She couldn't have understood, ask her again.'

By her tone I could tell the interpreter was doing her best, but in the end she admitted defeat.

'I'm sorry, she seems confused. I can't get her to tell me.'

She hadn't had a contraction in our presence, so I decided to get her in the ambulance and try quizzing her again on the way to hospital. Picking up an overnight bag, which was packed and ready by the door, I spoke briskly.

'Shall we go then?'

The interpreter put this to the woman and after another debate she turned back to me.

'She says she can't walk.'

'She can't walk? Why not?'

'I don't know.' The neighbour seemed embarrassed. 'She won't say.'

I heaved a sigh. Women in labour generally don't have a problem walking between contractions; there had to be more to all this, but for the life of me I couldn't think what it might be.

'Does she have an urge to bear down, or push?' I asked.

A few more words passed between them.

'She doesn't know.'

We can only work on what we see and, just as importantly, what we're told. It's not exactly an infallible system, but as examining a woman without good cause is out of the question it's the only system we have. Getting involved in a hands-on way only happens when there's little doubt that the birth is imminent, and by that stage most women would be grateful even if it were King Kong giving them a hand. Even Steve, with all his experience, was baffled, and decided to err on the side of caution and fetch our carry chair. While he was gone I spoke to the interpreter again.

'Could you ask her to sit down on the sofa while we're waiting, please.'

The neighbour passed on the request but the woman remained on her feet. I tried to keep the exasperation out of my voice.

'What's wrong? Why won't she sit down?'

'She says that she can't sit down.'

'Tell her to lie down then.'

'She can't lie down either.'

Whether she stood or sat didn't really matter, but her lack of compliance was testing my patience. Something had to be wrong, and there was more to it than the language barrier. More forcibly this time, the interpreter again asked her to sit down. She hesitated, then, with obvious reluctance, she shuffled towards the sofa. As she turned I was met by a sight that lives with me still. Just below her bottom was a large, swaying bulge in her culottes.

Steve came back with the chair and stopped in his tracks.

'My God! She's delivered!'

'No,' I said quickly. 'Nothing's happened while you've been out, I swear it. She must have had it before we got here.'

I felt sick; there hadn't been a sound from the baby

in the time we'd been in the room, which to my mind meant only one thing. Trying to keep a lid on the panic we both felt, we cajoled her into a half-kneeling position on the sofa and unceremoniously pulled down her culottes. What we saw made us catch our breath. Hanging from her, like a huge bean, was the intact caul, or fetal membrane, inside which was the baby and all the fluids. I'd never heard of such a thing even being a possibility, and I stared down in wonder at the sight of the baby through the misty membranes.

The woman shifted on to her side, and with little in the way of conscious thought I tried to break the membranes and release the baby. This was rather like trying to burst a taut balloon full of water and it took several attempts before I managed to make a tear and the fluids gushed out. The membrane collapsed about the baby and as I peeled it from his head he sucked in air and let out a cry that lifted my heart.

Steve went back out to radio for a midwife while I cleaned and wrapped the infant in a sheet before placing him in his mother's embrace. Together they lay there, the baby snuffling and gnashing his gums, while she looked on from an inscrutable face. I sat back and considered what had just happened. How, I wondered, could a woman give birth while standing up in the middle of the room and not feel moved to tell anyone? What had been going through her head?

As I thought over the sequence of events I recalled her first furtive glance at us when we walked in, and how she'd not looked in our direction again. It wasn't just a language barrier. She'd been alone and frightened out of her wits in an alien environment. She'd needed her family and they weren't there for her. Instead, she got Steve and me. I like to think that for most people we represent help, hope and reassurance, but there was no doubt in my mind that as far as she was concerned, we might as well have been a couple of Martians, and male ones to boot.

Chapter Nineteen

Our lack of success wasn't for want of trying. We'd done our best to establish some kind of rapport with the man, but so far he hadn't uttered a single word of sense. Larry pursed his lips and tried again.

'Come on! Give me a break, will you. Show me the cut on your hand and tell me what the bloody hell this is all about. I want to help you, but how can I if you won't speak to me properly?'

The man looked up from the rain-drenched pavement and for a second I thought Larry might be making some headway. But his reply took us back to square one.

'You want to help me? If you truly want to help me, then go and tell her that I love her! Tell her that I love her with all my heart. I know she would love me if only they would allow her to!'

'What the hell are you going on about?' Larry's voice was showing the strain. 'Who are "they"?'

'Her brothers! Who else? Go and tell them to let me speak to her. My hand means nothing, I would cut it off for her!'

He was Asian, in his early thirties and, it has to be said, cut a rather unprepossessing figure. His undoubtedly expensive suit had probably fitted him at some time in the past but it was now two sizes too small, so that his body resembled a randomly squeezed tube of toothpaste. His heavily oiled hair was slicked back and oozed well past his collar, which was held tightly in place by a pencil-thin red tie. Larry muttered something under his breath and gave him a long stare while he considered what to say next.

'I'm not going to stand round here all night! For the last time, let me see your hand!'

The plump, tear-stained face looked up again. 'I love her . . .'

'I don't know what you're talking about,' Larry snapped back in exasperation.

'No, I don't suppose you do. But that comes as little surprise to me. Is an artist ever really understood?'

Larry could only stare back.

Our present tactics clearly weren't working so we decided to change tack and try humouring him. If we could gain his confidence, maybe we could sort out his hand and then get on with the rest of the night's work. With this in mind I took over from Larry.

'So you love her, do you?'

'Yes! With every fibre of my being I love her!'

'But she doesn't love you.'

'How can she love me? She doesn't know me. All she knows of me are my songs.'

I faltered at the first hurdle. 'Your songs?'

'Yes, I come here often and sing for her. That's her room over there, where the light is on.' He pointed at a house across the street.

'Don't tell me you stand and sing under her window,' Larry said.

The man looked pained. 'What else can I do? Her family won't let me near her.'

'Doesn't she mind?' I asked.

'Of course not!' he said indignantly. 'Her brothers do though, and so does her father. Oh, her father! He is a terrible man. There is not one ounce of humanity beating in his chest.' As an afterthought he added, 'He does not like me one little bit. He shouts terrible things at me, but he doesn't understand that I have to express myself in song.'

'How did your hand come to be cut?' I asked the question while raising his hand and at last getting a close look at it.

'It was one of her brothers. He came running out of the house waving a knife like a bloody lunatic and shouting at me to go away. He said I was driving him mad! Maybe he *was* mad because he came very close with the knife and cut my hand.'

'You didn't go away though, did you?' I said as I bandaged the hand.

'No, but I considered it prudent to stop singing. You never know with people like that.'

The patient's name was Abdul and the cut on his hand, though by no means serious, did need a few stitches. I suggested that he should come to hospital with us and get it seen to. He was reluctant until Larry pointed out that it might be the girl's father who came out next. This thought made Abdul reflect carefully.

'Yes, that is a real possibility I am sure. Maybe I will come with you. It would be wise to have my hand looked at.'

With the decision made, he stood up and followed us to the ambulance. It was my misfortune to be the attendant that evening and Larry had already decided he was going to make the most of it. He settled himself in the driver's seat and, as we pulled away, he turned his head and shouted through to the back.

'Hey Abdul, do you think we could hear one of your songs?'

Abdul's eyes lit up. 'No, no, you don't want to hear my singing . . . do you?'

'Yes, of course we do. Go on, give us a song!' It was a mischievous act, but it wasn't aimed at Abdul: it was aimed squarely at me.

'Well, if you really want me to, I will start with my favourite.'

A look of intense concentration spread over his face as he straightened his back and squared his shoulders. His eyes flicked shut and after making some grotesque noises in an unsuccessful attempt to clear his throat, he seemed ready. This, I realized later, was my opportunity to nip things in the bud, but the moment passed when Abdul burst into life with all the vigour of someone who'd been kicked in the small of the back by a mule. His eyes snapped open, his head jerked back and he let out the most frightful high-pitched howl. It had to be a joke. Surely nobody could make such an awful noise and expect to be taken seriously. There was no melody, no rhythm; in fact there weren't even any detectable notes or words, just a prolonged cacophony of sound blasted out at full volume.

My initial reaction of confused amusement didn't last long. Amusement quickly turned to disbelief. Disbelief then turned to consternation as it dawned on me that Abdul was not only deadly serious, but clearly had no intention of stopping. Under the sustained barrage my resolve to humour him dissolved, leaving me with the problem of how to bring the noise to an end. Shouting at him while he was in the middle of a song would be rude but, as there was no way of telling when one song ended and the next began, there didn't seem to be any other way. I endured the racket for what must have been the best part of five minutes before taking the bull by the horns. Startled by the vehemence in my own voice, I shouted at him to stop. It had no effect. Eyes closed, and grimacing horribly as he worked his way round what I can only assume was a particularly tricky passage, he held up his bandaged hand as though fending off unwanted praise.

I looked from Abdul to the real villain of the piece. He was hunched forward over the steering wheel laughing quietly to himself, and there's no doubt he would have enjoyed it even more if he'd known that, apart from sounding like a rutting elk with laryngitis, Abdul also suffered from as bad a case of halitosis as I've ever encountered. Not to put too fine a point on it, his breath smelled as if it were being fanned over the decomposing corpse of a warthog. Restricted by the confines of the ambulance, it was simply horrible. If I'd been inclined to consider which was worse, his breath or his singing, it would have been too close to call.

When he abruptly stopped of his own volition I was caught off guard and, for want of anything else to say, I came out with 'Thank you.' I was of course thanking him for stopping, but he didn't see it that way. His eyes turned to slits and I could see every one of his gleaming white teeth as a huge smile flooded his face.

'You liked it? You really liked it? I have many more, I can also sing in English too . . . Listen.'

My protests were drowned out by the opening verse of 'Heartbreak Hotel'. If I'd made any allowances (and I'm not sure I had) for the fact that he'd so far been singing in his own language, they were now banished and I began to marvel at the restraint shown by the brother with the knife.

Meanwhile, Larry had been making suspiciously slow progress towards the hospital. What should have been a ten-minute journey looked as if it was going to take more like fifteen. This was to change when Abdul moved seamlessly into a mind-boggling rendition of 'Ain't Nothing But A Hound Dog'. On hearing it, Larry slammed shut the communicating door and his driving suddenly took on a sense of urgency. I had little choice but to sit out the remainder of the trip trying not to breathe while listening to a tone-deaf Elvis impersonator irredeemably ruining some songs I'd always liked. It was only when we reached the hospital that Abdul brought the concert to an end and I could make a bolt for the door.

I tried to catch Larry's eye as we made our way into Casualty but he was having none of it, and avoided my look while maintaining an extremely annoying grin on his face. We found the triage nurse at her desk and waited for her to finish riffling through some papers before presenting Abdul to her.

'Hi, this is Abdul. He's got a knife cut to his hand that might need a few stitches.'

'Oh, how did that happen?'

'Well . . .'

Abdul seized his chance before I could say any more and, pushing his face close to the nurse's, indignantly launched into a description of the circumstances of the assault and the unfairness of it all.

'It is the most foul luck! Why did fate decree that I should fall in love with a woman who is encumbered with such unreasonable and hostile brothers?'

The suggestion of a welcoming smile on the nurse's face was cruelly curtailed by the awful waft of his breath. She leaned back in her chair as discreetly as she could and, to her credit, did her best to remain impassive, but her frozen expression told its own story. Then, to my disbelief, Larry was at it again.

'Why don't you let the nurse hear one of your songs, Abdul?'

'Oh no . . . she is a busy lady. She wouldn't want to listen to me . . . would she?'

I recognized the tone of voice and looked daggers at Larry while the nurse tried to fend Abdul off.

'That would be nice,' she said, 'but not just now. Maybe later if we have a bit more time.'

Abdul took this as his cue and drew a deep breath. Larry, I noticed, was already halfway to the exit and I thought it might be wise to join him. We were almost at the door when the tortured strains of 'My Way' ripped through Casualty. I looked back to see Abdul standing with his arms flung out and his eyes closed, bellowing. The nurse was on her feet, glaring after us with an expression a voodoo priestess would have been proud of.

On the way back to the Street I tried to remonstrate with Larry, but it was water off a duck's back. He dismissed it all with a shrug.

'You've got to have a laugh now and again in this bloody job or you'd go nuts. Talking of having a laugh, I've set up something to get my revenge on H.'

'Revenge? What for?'

'What for? Just that little matter of him dropping a set of false teeth in my curry!'

'But he was getting his revenge on you for the snooker balls, wasn't he?' I protested.

'Yeah, but don't forget he tied a kipper to my engine before that.'

'So this is never going to stop?'

'Maybe this time it will, because he won't have a clue who's set him up. You're the only one to know it was me.'

I didn't like the sound of this. 'Look, don't include me in your plans.'

'OK. Just keep an eye on H when he scans the noticeboard. It should be good fun.'

When we got back to the Street, Mike was sixty points ahead of H on the snooker table. Larry waited with folded arms until H was lining up what should have been an easy pot, and then said loudly, 'I've seen those missed!'

His timing was perfect. The white ball skidded off the red and straight into the middle pocket. Howard smiled and lowered his cue.

'Good to see you back, Larry. Been busy out there looking after your drunken mates, have you?'

Larry smiled back.

'No, saving lives actually. But that's something you wouldn't know much about.'

'One thing I do know,' H replaced his cue in the

rack, 'the only time you ever manage to save a life is when you let someone else do the job—'

The exchange was cut short by the phone and as H walked over to answer it Larry said, 'He's in a good mood. He can't have seen the board yet.'

Two minutes later we were back on the road ourselves.

There can't be many people who've chased a suicidal man through a subterranean canal system at one o'clock in the morning. In fact, I wouldn't be surprised if Larry and I were the only people who ever have. It all started in a pub where the clientele regularly enjoyed after-hours drinking. The building was adjacent to a canal, which then passed under a four-lane city-centre road before re-emerging at a lower level some hundred yards away. It was a singularly dank, evil-smelling place and usually only frequented by creatures with four legs or more.

The case was described in somewhat ambiguous terms, leaving us unsure if someone had already committed suicide at the pub, or was about to. Several young men were waiting for us on the pavement when we turned into the street and one was in such an agitated state he jumped into our path flailing his arms like a windmill. Larry had to hit the brakes hard to avoid knocking him down and was still cursing when he emerged from his side of the ambulance and rounded on the culprit.

'You bloody idiot! You got a death wish or something?'

The young man was too busy shouting to listen. 'It's Ian! He's going to kill himself!'

'Judging by you, it must be contagious!' Larry snapped back. 'Now, get a grip of yourself. Who's Ian, and where is he?'

One of the other lads interrupted. 'Ian is Malcolm's lover . . . the guy you nearly ran over.'

The gay community was a good deal more clandestine back in the seventies, but if Larry was fazed by the answer he didn't show it.

'It's all my fault. If you want someone to blame, blame me!' Malcolm wailed.

'Nobody's blaming anybody for anything!' Larry tried to mellow his tone. 'Just tell us what's going on.'

'We were having a silly argument, you know what it's like after a few drinks, when all of a sudden Ian jumped up from the table and ran out saying he was going to end it all.'

'So he's not in the pub, he's run away?' I said.

'Yes, he's gone down to the canal!'

'Canal? What canal?' I'd no idea there was a canal anywhere near.

'It's down there.' Malcolm pointed a trembling finger to the shadows by the side of the pub where a rusty old gate hung from broken hinges. We crossed over and looked into the darkness below. After a moment I could make out a muddy path winding steeply down the embankment towards the dead water of the canal. I wasn't sure, but I thought I could hear muffled shouts drifting up on the night air.

'Is there someone else down there?' I asked.

'Just some of the lads from the pub. They're trying to stop Ian doing anything stupid,' Malcolm said.

Larry fetched a torch from the ambulance and we picked our way down to the towpath. Echoing voices came from the tunnel on our left and we carefully edged along the damp cobbles in their direction. Overhead electric lights were fixed to the roof but their ancient glass shades were so encrusted with grime and cobwebs that little light escaped. The murky illumination was just about enough to show us the way, and after about twenty feet the tunnel opened into a chamber containing a lock. It was a horrible place. The stagnant water gave off a fetid, cloying odour, which hung in the air and then crept over us like a chiffon shroud. The blue-brick walls glistened black with lichen and every few seconds a droplet of condensation fell from the roof to the inky water with an echoing plop. Rubbish lay in heaps all around and scuffling noises from the shadows indicated that our progress was not going unnoticed by the rats.

A group of young men were standing on our side of the canal shouting into the darkness opposite. I stared over, trying to catch sight of Ian in the shadows, then the light of Larry's torch picked him out squeezing up against a buttress. The celluloid image of Orson Welles in the sewers of Vienna jumped to mind, but quickly faded. Rather than Harry Lime's enigmatic smile greeting the beam of light, an indignant and petulant face confronted us. His opening words didn't come from the pen of a Hollywood scriptwriter either.

'Will you lot just piss off and leave me alone! If I want to die it's my business, not yours.'

His friends were trying to coax him back on to our side of the water. The tactics used ranged from ingratiating pleas to extravagant promises, and finally to threats of retribution when they got hold of him. The whole scenario perplexed me.

'Why don't you just go and grab him?' I asked the leader of the group.

'What! And spook him into throwing himself into the water?' He looked at me aghast. 'This needs careful negotiating. Charging across like bulls in a china shop might trigger a human tragedy.'

'It's not exactly Niagara Falls!' Larry said. 'It can't be more than three feet deep at most.'

As he spoke there was a clatter of shoes from the other side and we caught sight of Ian darting to a different buttress, shrieking as he went.

'Leave me alone, you bastards.'

It was plain that we could wait all night for his friends to resolve things, so Larry and I decided to cross the lock and bring Ian back. There wasn't a handrail on the slimy wooden walkway bridging the canal and I looked down with trepidation at old cans, oily duck feathers, bits of wood and various horribly organic-looking objects mummified in slicks of diesel fuel. As I've indicated before, there are times in the life of everyone working for the emergency services when they stop and reflect on their choice of career. For me, this was probably the first. What on earth was I doing here? Why was I under a Birmingham street in the middle of the night edging my way across a stinking canal while being watched by a sizeable group of inebriated young men? Sensible people were at home tucked up in bed – why wasn't I? Whichever way you looked at it, it was a perfectly good question.

With the rapidly fading torch beam casting grotesque shadows, we stepped off the gantry on the far side and made our way over the cobbles towards Ian. With nowhere to go, he placed his hands on his hips and indignantly indicated that we weren't welcome.

'I thought I told you to piss off!'

Larry and I grabbed an arm each.

'Don't touch me, leave me alone!'

Technically, what we were doing was wrong; we have no right to grab anyone against their will but we wanted out of this place and his protests only served to make me tighten my grip. Deciding to join the melodramatic mood, Larry moved closer and spoke into his ear.

'See that water?'

'Yes.'

'I sincerely hope you don't expect me, or anyone

else for that matter, to fish you out if you fall in.'

'I don't know what to expect. I can't think straight. You're hurting my arm.'

'Well, let me make it perfectly clear for you.' Larry stared him in the eye. 'If you fool around and end up in there, one of two things will happen. You'll either drown, or pick up some disease that will make the Black Death look like a mild case of chickenpox.'

Ian considered Larry's words. Then, with the air of someone who'd just been robbed of the chance to fulfil his destiny, he whispered, 'You win. Take me back.'

We frogmarched him across the gantry to his friends, where he fell emotionally into Malcolm's arms. It had all been a grand gesture that had then been enthusiastically taken up by his friends, who, I'm sure, secretly enjoyed every moment. They crowded round him, patting him on the shoulders and begging him never to do such a silly thing again. Larry and I, forgotten amid the rejoicing, were left to watch as the group made its way out of the tunnel, their excited voices fading eerily into the gloom. We followed at a distance. The torch had expended the last of its energy, returning the canal tunnel to the safe keeping of the denizens of the night.

Larry seemed keen that I shouldn't mention Abdul or Ian to the others when we got back as it would only give H more ammunition to use against him. He was already seen by most in the depot as a champion of drunks and lost causes, and it was a reputation he wanted to bring to an end. On this occasion he needn't have worried. Howard was the centre of attention when we walked into the room.

'Larry! Come and read this. I can't believe that even the idiots upstairs would pull a trick like this!' Howard pointed at a document printed on crested Metropolitan Ambulance Service paper in the centre of the locked, glass-fronted noticeboard. I craned over their shoulders and scanned down the lengthy proclamation.

It was headed 'Fitness for the Future' and was apparently addressing a deep concern felt by senior management over the health and general well-being of the road staff. There were a couple of tedious paragraphs on the organization's commitment to patient care being jeopardized if the workforce delivering that care wasn't at the peak of fitness itself. Then came the sting. Two weeks from the time of writing, anyone deemed to be overweight would be taken off front-line work and placed on light duties, which included delivering stores, stocktaking and washing vehicles. If their weight problem hadn't been addressed three months later, then redundancy would have to be considered. On a separate sheet of paper was a table laying out the optimal and maximum weights in relation to an individual's height.

Larry whistled. 'It makes you wonder what the bastards will come up with next. You must be pretty near the weight for your height, H.'

'Near it! I'm two stone over! What right have they to

tell me what I should weigh? And how the hell can anyone lose two stone in two weeks?'

'So what are you going to do?' Larry asked.

'I'm going to get the union on to it for a start.'

'He's already phoned Colin May for advice,' Steve chipped in.

'And what did he have to say?' Larry asked.

'He said it was half past one in the morning and to piss off.'

Larry couldn't suppress a grin. 'That's union reps for you. Just like policemen, they're never there when you need them.' Then, changing the subject slightly, 'What about Mike, surely he's over the weight limit too.'

Howard waved an arm towards the notice.

'You didn't read the final sentence. It says that anyone over fifty is exempt. And, get this ... all officers are exempt as well! It's unbelievable! I tell you what, this is going to end up in court.' Howard paused for breath and another thought struck him. 'Who are they to say I'm overweight anyway? I'm just big-boned.'

Steve looked at him sceptically.

'If that's the case, H, those bones in your arse must be one hell of a size.'

Howard didn't let the subject drop for the rest of the night, making each ring of the emergency phone seem like a heaven-sent means of escape. Our next case involved an elderly man who'd got up in the night to use the toilet and fallen, fracturing his hip. I waited until we were returning to station before tackling Larry about the 'height–weight chart'. He told me proudly how some time ago he'd discovered a way of getting into the boss's office without leaving a trace. This closely guarded secret gave the shift access to every scrap of correspondence passing across the boss's desk, something that came in very handy from time to time.

He'd used his skills the night before to spirit away some headed notepaper and a spare key to the notice-board. Later, at home, he drew up the document on a typewriter and surreptitiously slipped it on to the noticeboard when he came on duty. Then it was just a matter of sitting back and waiting. When I compli-mented him on the convincing way he'd worded it, he was dismissive.

'When you've been reading that kind of crap for a few years it's not difficult to imitate it. Come to think of it, I'd make a pretty good officer. All they seem to do is sit around in meetings and come up with rubbish.'

When seven o'clock came we were all lined up wait-ing to go home – all, that is, but Howard. He'd announced earlier he intended to wait until eight and have it out with the boss the moment he came in. What happened then, I heard from the day shift the following evening. It seems Howard was as good as his word and began berating the boss as he got out of his car. A heated exchange followed, which the boss tried to end by stalking off through to his office. H stuck close on his tail, and could be heard threatening to call all the union chiefs from London to Liverpool and arrange a petition of all the ambulance personnel in the country. The boss kept saying he didn't know what the hell H was talking about and that he should 'shut the fuck up' before he landed himself in trouble.

In the face of repeated denials and counter-denials of the document's existence, the two men finally strode down to the messroom and across to the noticeboard. Heaven only knows what went on in H's mind when his eyes fell on the empty space previously occupied by the infamous piece of paper. The blinding realization that he'd not only been set up, but also hung out to dry in a very public way, must have cut to the core of his being. If the day-workers were to be believed, and I have no reason to doubt them, he looked like a beached cod desperately searching for a way of drowning himself.

Chapter Twenty

The idea that our lives follow a predestined path is outrageous, so why do so many of us readily grasp the notion of fate? Why do we want to believe in a concept that's so plainly ridiculous? Maybe it's comforting to imagine that the Sword of Damocles doesn't choose its victims quite so randomly after all, and that fate has already decided when the sword should fall. Or perhaps deep in all of us there's a need to try and rationalize events we have no control over, so we see fate as a way of explaining the inexplicable.

My first year in the ambulance service concentrated my mind on such things. I suppose it's difficult to differentiate between fate and luck, but if for convenience' sake we call it luck then I saw a fair bit of it in that first year or so, good and bad. And I don't mean the kind of luck that happens every day to someone somewhere, like a knife missing an artery by a millimetre. I mean extraordinary luck or, as in this first case, an extraordinary lack of it.

The man was in a bus station and as he looked around there couldn't have been anything to suggest to him that he was only seconds away from a sudden, violent death. Had he been in a car, or on a train, or been crossing the road, he would have been aware of a risk but, as it was, his surroundings offered no conceivable threat. Sipping a coffee, he had wandered towards a pedestrian area well away from the bus lanes, which also provided a good vantage point for watching the comings and goings of the buses. The spot he'd chosen was raised about eighteen inches above the garage floor. Behind him was a wall, and a few feet in front were stout iron railings designed to prevent the unwary traveller from stumbling down the short drop.

So there he was, quietly minding his own business in unarguably the safest spot in the garage, when a bus entered the depot from the far end. It had a clear sixty yards to travel before reaching its bay and was apparently moving slowly towards its parking slot when it suddenly, and unaccountably, picked up speed. It continued accelerating towards the far wall and must have been travelling at over twenty miles an hour when it hit the raised area where our man was standing. There was an explosion of fibreglass as the front of the bus disintegrated, people dived in all directions to escape – but the man with the coffee had no chance. He was in the bus's direct line. The vehicle smashed into the wall taking the railings and the man with it, killing him instantly.

For me, the case was made all the more poignant by the fact that the man had done nothing to deserve such a fate. It was sheer unmitigated bad luck, a classic case of being in the wrong place at the wrong time. Why the bus careered out of control remained a mystery to me. I scoured the local press for a report of the inquest but never found one.

As with the man at the bus station, some people suffer the most appalling luck when others seem to have all the good luck in the world. Take the Houdini-like escape made by a car driver who I'd say, at the risk of mixing my metaphors, used up all his nine lives in one go. He was driving out of Birmingham on an urban expressway towards Spaghetti Junction. This junction, as its name suggests, is a sprawling tangle of motor-ways, which offers plenty of opportunities for an inattentive driver to make mistakes. Our driver had already missed the M6 turn-off, and shortly after realizing this was confronted with another choice of exits. He took too long trying to decide between the two alternatives and ended up taking an unlikely third route, which was to drive at sixty miles an hour into the crash barrier dividing them.

The first five or six feet of the crash barrier rises from ground level at an angle of about thirty degrees then runs horizontally at a height of three feet parallel with the carriageway. It was this angled section that launched his car into the air like a Harrier Jump Jet from the deck of an aircraft carrier. His car shot up and struck the underside of the motorway running above, then fell back to earth nose first, smashing into the ground with considerable force.

Steve and I arrived to find the car concertinaed to half its length with the engine sitting in what was left of the driver's seat. Several other vehicles had stopped and their occupants were hanging about watching from a safe distance. One man was standing on his own a little closer to the wreck, holding a cigarette.

'Don't even think about lighting that!' Steve said as we walked past him. 'Can't you smell the petrol?'

'Oh, sorry.' The man was contrite. 'I wasn't going to light it, I'm just a bit shook up by this, sorry.'

Ignoring him, and aware of the tight knot of tension building in the pit of my stomach, I knelt down and peered into the wreck. What was once the front seating area was now a chaotic mass of mangled metal, the only immediately recognizable object being part of the twisted steering wheel. I shifted my position slightly and, trying to ignore the sickly stench of petrol and hot oil, looked again. There was no sign of the driver.

It didn't make sense. Nobody could have escaped. An agile kitten would have been hard pressed to find the space to turn round in there. To the background ticking of cooling steel I searched again for signs of the occupant, but there was no doubt about it: the car was empty. Mystified, I straightened up and looked over at Steve, who was checking from the other side. He looked back and shrugged.

The bystander with the cigarette had been looking over my shoulder as I scanned the wreckage and felt moved to comment.

'It's a right bloody mess, isn't it?'

'Yes,' I said curtly, before pointedly moving away from him and walking round the car to peer in from different angles. Undaunted, he followed close behind and I was about to suggest he should get back in his car and continue his journey, when he said, 'There's nobody in there.' Then, almost by way of an after-thought, 'I was on my own.'

I turned and looked at him properly for the first time. He was a short man; slightly overweight perhaps, but otherwise he looked fit and well. His clothes were neat and tidy, without rips or blemishes.

'Let me get this straight,' I said. 'You're telling me you were in this car?'

'Well, yes. I was driving it actually.' He appeared almost apologetic.

I looked again at the vehicle and then back at him with the feeling that I'd missed something important.

'You couldn't have been! I mean . . . were you thrown out before the crash?'

'No, I climbed out before you got here.'

'You're going to have to start from the beginning,' I said.

His memory of events was rather blurred, but it seemed that after striking the underside of the motor-way the car had flipped over. He had a vague impression of tumbling about inside before an almighty bang signalled the vehicle's return to earth. When everything was quiet, he tried to open his eyes and move but found that his face was pressed into what felt like a mound of cushions. There was a moment's panic when he thought he was being suffocated but, after a struggle, he managed to turn his head to one side and take in a gulp of air. He found himself jammed in the back-seat footwell surrounded by the protective upholstery of the seats. He lay for a minute testing each limb while he got his breath. Everything worked, so he climbed out through the gap where the rear window had been and emerged without a mark on him, not even a bruise. He finished his story by coming out with what must have been the understatement of the year.

'I've been lucky, I suppose.'

'Lucky? I'll say you were lucky.' I looked back at the smashed car. 'I've never seen anything like it. You obviously weren't wearing your seat belt.'

'No. I don't believe in them. If I'd had it on . . . well, it doesn't take much working out where I'd be now.' He held up his cigarette. 'I don't suppose you've got a light, have you?'

I was working with Howard one night when an extraordinary event took place that still has me scratching my head and wondering if there really is such a thing as fate. If there is, then that night it chose between two teenage lads sitting side by side in a stolen car.

They'd taken the vehicle from a car park in the city centre and were heading out of town at high speed when they came to grief. By chance a policeman was parked up eating a sandwich when the stolen car flashed past and went straight through a red light without slowing down. At almost the same moment another car entered the junction from the left. Fate must have had something else in store for the occupants of this second vehicle. If they'd been so much as one second further into their journey, just five feet further down the road, they would have been hit broadside and the result would have been carnage. As it was, the stolen car passed a hair's breadth in front of them doing about sixty miles an hour.

The youths almost got away with it, but it wasn't to be. The bumper of the second car touched the rear bumper of the stolen vehicle with just enough force to send it spinning wildly out of control across the road, where it struck a kerb that launched it sideways through the air. It demolished a bus shelter before being well nigh cut in half by a lamp post. Even then there was still enough momentum remaining in what was left of the car to send it rolling and spinning on down the road, bouncing off parked cars and walls as it went.

Howard and I arrived six or seven minutes later, to be met by a sight that beggared belief. On the far side of the junction there was a trail of twisted and torn metal extending for at least a hundred yards. At first there didn't seem to be any central point to the mayhem, nothing to focus on that might give us a clue as to what had happened. Then I spotted the rear end of a car sitting like an abandoned handcart on the pavement. It was barely recognizable; all that was left was a pair of wheels and the boot. We've all seen mangled cars on television or in real life, but I'd never seen a vehicle that had more or less disintegrated on impact as this one had. The whole area was like a scrap yard. Everywhere we looked was just a jumble of doors, body panels, seats and bits of engine. Standing some way off in the middle of the mayhem was the solitary figure of the policeman.

With the sirens of other emergency vehicles growing louder in the distance, we picked our way through the debris to join him. He was clearly shaken, having witnessed the accident, but his lack of colour was as nothing in comparison to the lad sitting nearby on the pavement. He didn't look so much as if he had seen a ghost, but more as if he was the ghost himself. He really did seem to be in deep shock. Maybe he'd managed to avoid the flying debris by the skin of his teeth as he passed by and now the reaction was setting in.

'Are you going to be OK?' I asked him.

Without looking up he mumbled a reply. 'Yeah, yeah . . . I'm fine.'

I turned back to the policeman as H was asking him about the number of casualties.

'There was two of them in the car. The other one's

up the road a bit.' The officer pointed in the direction of what looked like a body under a blanket some forty feet away.

'So where's the other body?' Howard asked.

'Other body? I told you, there were only two of them. There's that one,' he jabbed his finger again towards the shape under the blanket, and then turned and nodded at the lad sitting at our feet. 'And this one.'

It hadn't crossed my mind that the youth might have been in the car, and by the look on H's face it hadn't crossed his either.

'Have you moved him?' Howard asked as he crouched down beside the lad and began examining him for injuries.

'No. I think this is where he ended up. It's where I found him anyway.' The policeman lowered his voice and looked back up the road. 'That one certainly isn't going to move anywhere, he's a right mess. I thought it best to put a blanket over him.'

'I'd better go and have a look,' I said, and leaving H to his examination I started to crunch my way over the sea of broken glass and metal sheeting that had once been the bus shelter.

The policeman was at my side giving me a vivid description of the accident when I noticed something organic-looking smeared on the pavement. Under the streetlights it was a yellow-grey colour and could have been anything, but I had an uncomfortable feeling that I knew what it was. We took another few steps and my suspicions were confirmed. Mingling with the acid leaking from an upturned car battery was an unmistakable mound of human brain bigger than my fist. I stopped in my tracks. With a good bit more than half his brain spread down the road, the lad under the blanket didn't stand a chance. Never having been one for dwelling on the more ghoulish side of the job, I had no wish to subject myself to the sight, so I returned to help H.

He was still crouched over his patient and looked up at me.

'I can't find anything wrong with him, not a bloody thing! How can he be thrown out of a car at that speed and just have a few scratches?' He stood up and came closer. 'It doesn't make sense. His chest's clear and he's not complaining of any neck or head pain.'

I thought back to the child we'd taken from the back of the car a few weeks previously.

'No abdominal tenderness?' I asked.

'Nothing at all.' He leaned a little closer. 'I take it the other one's had it?'

I nodded. We busied ourselves for the next few minutes carefully immobilizing the youth while he lay silently accepting all that was happening to him. He didn't ask any questions and, when replying to ours, he restricted his answers to the bare minimum. His lack of any recognizable injuries presented H with a dilemma that I don't think he'd faced before. Should he ask me to radio ahead and alert the hospital staff that we were coming, even though we couldn't find anything wrong with the patient? It seemed perverse but in the end he decided that we'd better take the lad in, based purely on the fact he'd been hurled out of a crashing car at up to sixty miles an hour.

As I pulled away from the kerb a second ambulance arrived to deal with the body. Howard kept a close eye on our patient during the short trip to hospital and with the help of some oxygen he seemed to perk up. His colour improved and he started asking questions, a few of which I could hear from the driver's seat.

'Where's Trev?'

'Trev? Was he the lad in the car with you?' Howard asked.

'Yeah. Is he OK?'

'I don't know. Another ambulance crew is looking after him.' It was a lie of course, and H quickly changed the subject. 'Were you driving?'

'Driving what?'

'The car. You've been in a car crash, don't you remember?'

'Oh yeah, sort of. Where's Trev?'

And so the conversation continued in circles until we reached the hospital.

The Casualty consultant and a couple of nurses were waiting for us at the doors, and as we unloaded the stretcher Howard launched into a brief account of what had happened, plus his observations of the patient's condition.

'He was in the front seat of a car that crashed into a lamp post at high speed. The car was completely wrecked and he was flung out. We found him sitting in the road.' H carried on talking as we pushed the stretcher down the corridor. 'His obs are OK and he doesn't complain of any pain. He's got full limb movement but he's showing signs of concussion. I can't find any trace of a head injury though.'

We were now in the resuscitation room and lifting the patient across on to the hospital trolley.

'Was he wearing a seat belt?' the consultant asked. H was taken aback for a moment.

'I don't know, I didn't ask him.'

'It's important.'

'Yes, but as he can't even remember if he was driving or not, I didn't think it was particularly relevant.'

'Not relevant?'

'I can't have explained very well just how serious an accident this was. The car was smashed to pieces and he was thrown out. The seat he was sitting in is probably in someone's front garden and the belt wrapped round a tree fifty yards away.'

The consultant sniffed and, thrusting his stethoscope into his ears, listened intently to the patient's chest before moving round to examine his neck and spine.

I was aware of Howard's frustration but the consultant's scepticism was understandable as the patient in front of him had less in the way of injuries than you'd expect of someone who'd fallen off a push-bike. A nurse came into the cubicle and waited for the consultant to finish his initial checks before addressing him in lowered tones.

'Another ambulance has turned up. The crew want someone to come and certify their patient as deceased.'

'Is it the other one from the same accident?'

'Yes, I believe so,' she said, taking care not to be overheard.

'OK, I'll be out in a moment.'

When he returned from viewing the broken remains he wore a thoughtful expression as he beckoned Howard over.

'They were both sitting in the front of the same car?'

'Yes, side by side.'

'It's hard to believe – incredible in fact.' The doctor shook his head. 'I doubt if I've seen worse injuries. Tell me again about the crash.'

Now he had an attentive listener, H went over it all again and by the time we pushed our stretcher out of the room the medical team had begun what was going to be a meticulous re-examination of the lad.

It must have been an hour later when we found ourselves back in Casualty and went looking for news of the lad. The consultant was holding open the resuscitation-room door as a porter pushed out a trolley with the patient on it. As the porter headed off in the direction of the wards, Howard spoke to the doctor.

'Did you find anything wrong with him in the end?'

The doctor released the door and watched it swing back and forth for a moment.

'Nothing, absolutely nothing. We've gone over him from head to toe twice. A few bruises here and there, he'll be sore in the morning, but that's about it. We're going to monitor him for twenty-four hours, but I'm sure he'll be OK. I still don't understand how two people can be sitting, what, six inches apart, and one is smashed to hell while the other comes out virtually untouched. It really is remarkable.'

'Fate?' Howard suggested.

'Yes,' said the doctor. 'For want of a better explanation, I think we'll have to put it down to fate.'

Chapter Twenty-one

There were two vacancies on the shift when I joined. I don't know for sure why the other wasn't filled sooner, but I have a sneaking suspicion it might have had something to do with new recruits not wanting to set foot anywhere near Henrietta Street. Whatever the reason, I had to wait nine months before news came through that the remaining vacancy was at last being filled. I was delighted that my status as general dogsbody and tea maker was coming to an end. Life at the bottom of the pecking order hadn't been easy, and I have to confess to feeling a certain amount of sadistic pleasure at the thought of someone else taking on the role.

When he was due in for the first time I slumped into one of the messroom chairs in preparation for his entrance and adopted what I fancied to be a studied, devil-may-care attitude. My plan was to ignore him as he crept through the door and let him stew for a bit before casting him a nod and as neutral a 'hello' as I could manage. I would then declare how bored I was and turn to one of the others and suggest a game of Scrabble. If that didn't impress him, I might wish out loud for a decent crash on the M6 to liven things up a bit. (Something I'd yet to attend, and dreaded with a passion.) But, to use the words of the Scottish bard, 'the best laid schemes o' mice an' men gang aft a-gley'.

The moment Jack Turner strode into the room I knew my tea-making days weren't over just yet. He must have been a good ten or twelve years older than me and had the relaxed, purposeful air of someone blissfully untroubled by self-doubt or worry. He was well built in a fleshy kind of way, with large hands and a rounded face featuring a bulbous nose one size too big. In saying that, it was a friendly, cosy face. A face, as I was to learn much later, that brought out the motherly instincts in any woman it chose to smile upon.

I watched with a sinking heart as he came over and confidently introduced himself before indicating the cluttered chair next to mine and asking if it were free.

'Of course,' I said, and hurriedly cleared the pile of old newspapers. As I threw them on to the table it struck me that my eagerness to oblige had already compromised my laid-back persona. Using a casual tone, I tried to regain it. 'So, you're just out of training school, are you?'

'Yes. I finished last Friday. How long have you been on the job?'

This question put me firmly on the back foot. 'Well, let me think . . . it must be about nine months.'

'Oh, so you're pretty new yourself. Another three months before you qualify.'

Damn and blast. 'Yes,' I said, 'something like that.'

'I don't know how you felt when you started,' Jack continued, 'but I'm as nervous as hell. You blokes are going to have to nursemaid me for a bit.'

This was more like it, not that he looked very nervous to me.

Steve tapped out his pipe. 'Nothing to be nervous about. You're with me tonight. The time to worry is when you're crewed up with Larry.' Steve blew through his pipe and seemed to reconsider. 'No, that's not fair. If you want to learn the job properly, then Larry's probably the man to teach you.' Larry looked up suspiciously as Steve continued. 'Just watch everything he does and then make sure to do the exact opposite. That way you won't go far wrong.'

Larry pulled a face. 'Very funny. I'm the only professional on this shift of has-beens.'

I waited for Mike's reaction, but he didn't come out from behind his newspaper.

'What were you doing before this, Jack?' Larry asked.

'After leaving school I did ten years as a ladies' hairdresser . . .'

This time a pair of eyes did appear over the top of Mike's newspaper, and scrutinized Jack carefully.

'. . . then I did about seven years as a continental HGV driver. Since I gave that up I've been finding work as a freelance nightclub doorman.'

And that just about summed Jack up – contradictions at every turn.

When the conversation moved on to Jack's motives for joining the ambulance service he displayed an almost boyish perception of the job. He wanted a career to be proud of. He wanted to go home at night with the satisfaction of knowing that, in one way or another, his day had been well spent helping folk who weren't in a position to help themselves. All very laudable, but if anybody else on the shift held such romantic ideals they certainly hadn't voiced them when I was around. Jack didn't seem to notice the raised eyebrows and barely concealed smiles, and continued waxing lyrical on the joys of helping others until interrupted by the phone.

Larry took down the details and looked at me.

'We're going to a social club!'

I raised my eyes to the ceiling and let out a snort of irritation.

'Bloody social clubs . . . they should all be closed down!' As it happens, I don't like social clubs but, if I'm honest, my outburst was more designed to impress on Jack that I'd been around long enough to be as world-weary as anyone else on the shift.

'What's happening there?' Jack asked, sitting up in his seat.

Larry spoke over his shoulder as he pulled on his coat.

'Oh, I dunno, someone's collapsed or something.'

Jack looked concerned. 'That could be serious, couldn't it?'

Larry had reached the door by now and said, grudgingly, 'Yeah, I suppose so.'

'Good luck then.'

Larry hesitated a moment, then carried on out with me close behind.

Wishing someone good luck just wasn't done. In fact, any expression of encouragement, endearment, praise or even sympathy was looked on with suspicion, and brickbats, insults and sarcasm were the preferred methods of communication. Depending on the inflection in the voice, and facial expression of the speaker, an insult could be high praise indeed. Not being insulted or, even worse, being ignored were the real causes for concern. Steve saw it as his job to right Jack's wrong, and shouted after us, 'It's not that pair who need luck. It's the poor bloody patient who's going to need all the luck he can get!'

Jack might have had cause to reassess his new-found mission in life if he'd been there to see our patient. He was one of a surprisingly large number of people who, when all else has failed, see feigning illness as a legitimate way of drawing attention to themselves. Maybe these people were indulged as children and never saw the need to abandon a winning formula when they grew up. What they don't seem to realize is that they might fool the people they intended to fool, but seldom, if ever, will they fool an experienced ambulance crew. It's an aspect of our work I hadn't been forewarned about, and certainly hadn't anticipated. For that reason it deserves a mention as an example of what we have to contend with on a depressingly regular basis. On the plus side, it gives me the chance to express my loathing of social clubs.

It was towards the end of a busy Saturday night and the drink had been flowing freely all evening, leaving everyone in high spirits. A sudden commotion on the dance floor probably attracted little attention at first but when the music stopped and the lights came up, people started to worry about a man slumped on the floor. He was unconscious and, despite their best efforts, no one was able to rouse him. The general consensus among the onlookers was that if he wasn't already dead, he soon would be. His frantic wife fell to her knees and, clasping the limp body to her ample bosom, howled in desperation.

'Someone do something . . . someone call an ambulance!'

We arrived ten minutes later to find an elaborate chain of middle-aged men had been set up to guide us down the potholed drive to the club car park. The first link in the chain was out in the middle of the road waving us towards the entrance, and as we swung past him our headlights picked out more men strategically placed at ten-yard intervals to urge us onwards. Looking back through the rear-view mirrors I watched each peel off as we passed and start to trot after us. By the time we pulled up at the club entrance a faltering group of red-faced, pot-bellied men, each a potential patient in his own right, trailed in our wake. A fresh group ushered us into the building and we began to hear the first of many opinions about what might be wrong with the patient. Half listening to someone telling me he was pretty sure it had to be a subarachnoid haemorrhage, we crossed the foyer to the dance floor.

If you haven't had the pleasure of spending an evening in a social club, perhaps I should offer a brief description of what you're missing. Predominant among the clientele are family groups gathered round tables dragged together at the start of the evening. Positioned at the centre of the group, if they are lucky enough to have one, is the proverbial grandmother. She's been using the club for the past sixty years and sits behind an untouched glass of stout like a collapsed soufflé. She smiles and nods in a vaguely uncomprehending way as people pass by, not quite sure who they are or where she is. At her side sit her heirs apparent – the dutiful son and daughter-in-law.

Socially, this pair are in their prime. They're in their mid-fifties, have been coming to the club for thirty years and as a result know everybody and, more importantly, everybody knows them. The daughter-in-law assumed the mantle of group matriarch in a bloodless coup when her mother-in-law's erratic behaviour began to be an embarrassment. Her husband is her middle-aged bull. His jacket and tie were removed several hours ago when the heat started to get to him; he now sits glassy-eyed, looking flushed and hypertensive. He's wondering if he can manage to drink the three pints bought for him at last orders. His wife, gin and tonic in hand, and beads of sweat breaking through disintegrating make-up, laughs raucously at some bawdy remark. When she turns to her daughter-in-law to share the joke, the tight red dress she somehow managed to squeeze into hours earlier groans in protest as the rolling flesh beneath searches for a way of escape.

The matriarch's daughter and son-in-law represent the third generation. They're in their twenties and uncomplainingly accept a place on the periphery. The daughter has to stay sober and, hating every moment, sits tight-lipped nursing an orange juice. This isn't just because she's the driver; sobriety will come in handy later when she gets her husband home and has to steer him away from peeing in the wardrobe before settling him down for the night in the spare room. But that's still to come. At the moment he's ticking over nicely on a bellyful of beer and feels in fine fettle. He sees himself as the protector of the group and will have spent most of the evening on his feet patrolling the boundaries of their family space, checking everyone's glass is full and badgering them all into having a good time. If there's any sign of trouble he's ready and willing to rise to the occasion.

The only truly neutral ground is on the dance floor, which is usually occupied by children in party frocks trailing balloons in their wake as they jig around in time to Tom Jones. The other family groups are scattered around the main room. The different clans communicate by shouting across the aisles while taking care to maintain an unspoken but well-defined distance. A few rogue males prowl unchallenged among the tables. These unaccompanied men of indeterminate age don't have any defendable territory of their own and, as a result, are tolerated when they temporarily trespass into a dominant male's domain. He doesn't see them as a threat, and knows they will gravitate back to the bar when their glass is empty or, if everyone gets lucky, the Abba tribute band takes to the stage.

It was one of these rogue males who, his voice laden with sarcasm, shouted over as soon as he clapped eyes on us. 'Well, well, well. Look who's here!' Then, more menacingly, 'Where the bloody hell have you been?'

We ignored him and made our way towards the swaying buttocks of a woman kneeling over the collapsed man. She was shouting into his ear, pleading with him to wake up, while a couple of men vigorously fanned him with beer mats. The atmosphere hung heavy with stale smoke, beer and cheap aftershave.

'He could have died in the time it's taken you wankers to get here!'

The man at the bar had found his voice again.

One of the other single men sitting nearby tried to placate him, as if speaking to a child. 'Now, now, Jim. Leave them to get on with their job.'

Pint in hand, Jim slid heavily off his barstool and came forward, only to be intercepted by another drinker who put an arm round him and steered him back to the bar. An apologetic bar steward tried to make amends.

'Don't mind him. He's a great bloke really; it's just that he's had a few. You know what it's like.'

I looked warily across at Jim, now glowering at us over the top of a fresh pint as another voice shouted out, 'Are you two going to do something, for God's sake?'

With the threat seemingly lifted, we were able to get a look at the patient, whose name was Tom. He was flat on his back and seemingly unconscious. But was he really? Even in my short career I'd seen enough genuinely unconscious people to be suspicious of Tom. The messages the collapsed body sends out are varied. Some are obvious, some subliminal. In most unconscious people the mouth is open and the eyelids are often not fully closed. The breathing tends to be noisy and may be irregular, the skin takes on a different pallor and the limbs are arranged randomly. Muscle tone is reduced so there is little or no resistance when you lift, say, an arm. Tom had it all wrong. His mouth was firmly closed – it would look ungainly if it was hanging open – and his eyelashes were flickering. The arrangement of the limbs had a theatrical look: he'd done his best to make his pose dramatic but had over-done it, and one arm could only be in its position if consciously held there.

His wife, the owner of the swaying buttocks, was weeping uncontrollably as she leaned over, nuzzling his hair. Larry stepped closer and placed a gentle hand on her shoulder while suggesting she move back to allow him to check Tom's vital signs. She looked up at him from a mascara-streaked face, and wailed.

'He's my husband . . . and I love him.'

'Yes, I'm sure you do,' Larry said. 'But I can't do much while you're lying on top of him, can I?'

Reluctantly, she lurched to her feet and staggered into the arms of a woman friend.

Tom's eyes remained firmly shut, but when Larry brushed an eyelash with his finger the lid flickered noticeably. When your eyes are unexpectedly threatened it's impossible not to react in some way, though there's no such reaction in a genuinely un-conscious person. Larry decided to give Tom a chance to get out of the hole he was digging for himself and 'wake up' of his own accord. He told him quietly that the game was up and to stop wasting our time. This advice fell on stony ground, so the next thing to try was painful stimuli – an accepted way of checking someone's level of consciousness. Larry pressed a biro down on to the cuticle of a randomly selected finger-nail. Depending on the pressure applied, this can be very painful. Not many people can avoid reacting, but our man was made of sterner stuff than most and didn't flinch. Round one to him.

I'd come to learn there's always something behind this kind of behaviour, and looked about for someone to tell me what had happened before Tom's dramatic collapse. However, the picture I was initially given was of social harmony. Everyone, including Tom, had been having a great time and there'd been no unpleasantness of any kind.

'Are you sure there wasn't some sort of argument?' I persisted.

'There was something,' said a girl of about seventeen who'd appeared at my side. 'His wife was dancing a lot with some bloke and I don't think Tom liked it much.'

A man listening nearby grimaced as he suppressed a belch, then confirmed the story.

'That's right. Tom was getting pretty pissed off, especially when she kept looking over and kind of goading him.'

'And this was just before he collapsed?' I asked.

'Yes, I suppose it was.'

So there it was: cause and effect. Tom had decided that the only way to win back his wife's attention was to give her a fright by passing out.

By now the group of people gathered around Larry and Tom were getting restless.

'Do something! Give him some oxygen.'

'Take him to hospital!'

'He's not breathing. Are you just going to stand there and watch him die?'

Above their heads, Jim was shouting from the bar, 'I told you! They're just a pair of wankers!'

There seemed a real possibility we'd be lynched if we didn't get Tom on his feet quickly, or put him on our stretcher and rush him to hospital, which of course was exactly what he wanted. If we attempted to explain to his friends that Tom was conning them, that probably wouldn't have gone down too well either. Frustrated at the thought of Tom succeeding with his little game, I decided to have one more go at rousing him.

A few days earlier in Casualty I'd watched a doctor 'wake up' a patient who was playing dead. He'd gripped an area high up on the patient's Achilles tendon between forefinger and thumb and pinched hard. If the tirade of curses it elicited from the 'dead body' was anything to go by, it must have been very painful. I was hugely impressed by this example of the wonders of modern medicine and asked the doctor to show me the exact area to squeeze. Now was my chance to use this new skill, if only I could find the right spot. I bent over Tom and pulled up one of his trouser legs. Estimating where to pinch, I used all the pressure I could generate – and was instantly rewarded with a reaction as gratifying as it was explosive. He reared up and scrambled to his feet with an animal howl, fists clenched and eyes bulging.

'What bastard's trying to break my bastard leg!'

The people around fell silent as Tom glared at them in search of the culprit. Only then did it slowly dawn on him that he'd given the game away. His mouth opened and closed a couple of times as he raised the back of one hand to his brow. When he eventually found his voice it had a 'little boy lost' quality to it.

'Where am I? What's happening?'

Swaying dangerously, he took a couple of backward steps until he made contact with the chair someone had thoughtfully pushed into his path. He slumped on to it with a groan. I moved forward, pretending to take his pulse while asking with deep concern if there was anything else I could do for him. He gave me a long, hard look and, realizing I was the cause of his embarrassment, spoke in a low voice only I could hear.

'I'll tell you what you can do, pal. You can piss off!'

So that's what we did, and ten minutes later we were back at the Street.

If I'd been hoping Jack might nip into the kitchen and put the kettle on when we got back, I was to be disappointed. He was too busy entertaining the others with tales from his lorry-driving days. Mortified by the seeming ease with which he'd managed to ingratiate himself with the rest of the shift, I stomped off to make the tea, petulantly clattering things about in the kitchen as I did so. While I waited for it to infuse I could hear Jack talking about a prostitute he'd taken back to his lorry while on a stopover in Naples. He was a good storyteller and, despite myself, I couldn't help but smile as the others laughed.

I won't go into the detail of how he made the ghastly discovery that the attractive young lady was in fact a transvestite; suffice to say that Jack had everyone in stitches. The laughter continued as he went on to tell them how, after kicking the high-heeled hooker on to the street, he found his wallet was missing. Furious at his own gullibility, not to mention the loss of his money and papers, he woke a German lorry driver parked nearby and together they went into town to see if they could lay their hands on the thief. After trawling every back-street bar in Naples for six hours they returned to the lorry park with the dawn, empty-handed and so drunk there was nothing else for it but to crash into their bunks.

Mike couldn't resist chipping in. 'You'll never see thieves and pickpockets like the ones you get in Nairobi. Our barracks had to be nailed to the ground despite being patrolled twenty-four hours a day. The orders were to challenge, and fire on if necessary, anyone found inside the perimeter fence. When the locals got wind of the danger they sent their kids in, knowing we wouldn't dare shoot them. They stripped naked and smothered themselves in oil, so even if you did manage to get a hand on one of them he slipped out of your grasp like a wet eel. The little buggers could take the pillow from under your head and you'd know nothing about it till morning.'

'When I was out there they used to push a pole through the window with a hook and line attached like a fishing rod,' Steve said. 'It was no problem to lift a wristwatch off a locker from fifteen feet.'

'That's right,' Mike agreed. 'I'd forgotten about that. We had to sleep with the shutters bolted, which is no joke in Nairobi, I can tell you.'

And so, as usual, the conversation became an endless stream of anecdotes, this time on the topic of robbery and crime. One minute we were fighting off pickpockets in Port Said, and the next being warned of the perfidious nature of the fearsome Eban tribe of Borneo. (They apparently came from a proud lineage of headhunters, and had been drafted in by the British as bodyguards to the local dignitary.) When Jack took the floor to describe in graphic detail the trials of being locked up in a Yugoslavian police cell overnight after a bar fight, he held the attention of the room, including me. This was in spite of the umbrage I felt at the ease with which he'd won over everyone on the shift . . . and on his first night too! I'd have been quite startled then to be told that one day he'd be one of the best friends I had, on or off the service.

The conversation was brought to a halt when the nightclubs began to discharge their clientele on to the streets. Within a matter of minutes we were all out on the road. Larry and I were the lucky ones. Instead of joining the others in the delightful task of scraping up intoxicated youngsters, we were off to one of the more salubrious parts of the city. It was perhaps just as well, because I was still seething at the way Tom had flagrantly wasted our time at the social club, not to mention the abuse and implied threat of violence. But the job has a habit of lifting your spirits just as easily as it sometimes dampens them. The man we were going to help was from the opposite end of the spectrum to Tom. The place where he was staying wasn't exactly a social club either.

The high red-brick wall that ran for almost a hundred yards along the perimeter hid most of the building from view, but from the forest of Victorian chimney stacks peeking over the top it was clear that this wasn't your common or garden residence. The impression was reinforced when the heavy wrought-iron gates across the entrance swung open without any visible assistance – a common enough trick these days, but back then you only saw that kind of thing on *The Avengers*. In front of us, illuminated by lamps hidden among mature rhodo-dendrons, a gravel drive swept in an arc towards the kind of house most of us would expect to pay to visit. Larry let out a soft whistle as he drove in.

Waiting for us on the steps was a man in his late twenties dressed in a dark suit. He was tall with the lithe, powerful air of a sportsman, and the amiable smile of an old friend. He nodded us through into an oak-panelled reception hall where we waited as he secured the door. It was only when he turned to lead the way up the heavily carpeted staircase that I noticed the two-way radio held discreetly in his left hand.

'You were quick,' he said.

'Yes, we weren't too far away . . .'

'If you'll follow me I'll show you up. Chilly night, isn't it? Autumn's on the way all right.'

He rambled on about the weather as we followed him along the main landing. All we knew was that an elderly man had been suffering chest pains, and this chap, whoever he was, didn't seem inclined to enlighten us any further. I darted a mystified glance towards Larry, who returned the look without saying anything. Our guide stopped in front of an open door and ushered us through with another winning smile.

'Here we are. I'll be waiting out here if you need me.'

It was a spartan room by any standards. Just a few bits and pieces of oversized oak furniture were scattered around and, in the centre, an enormous double bed from where a little old man lay blinking at us. As the purpose of our visit, he should have commanded my full attention, but something else had caught my eye. Hanging from the wardrobe door op-posite was a garment I recognized immediately. Its deep magenta red seemed to shimmer magically against the neutral colour scheme. Attached to it by a cord, and looking like an old dishcloth, was a straw-coloured wig. There was no mistaking what I was looking at: it was a circuit judge's robe of office. The building had to be a hostel for judges, and the Milk Tray guy outside a Special Branch officer.

Unnerved, I looked back at the man in the bed. His white hair was tousled and, with the blankets drawn up to his chin, he gave the impression of someone hiding from the world. It's not every day you come across a judge tucked up in bed, and my thought processes seemed to clog up and stall. His elevated position in society shouldn't have made any difference to the way I approached him, but it did, and still I hesitated. Here was a man who, in his working life, wielded immense power, whose every word was listened to and weighed, a man whose cold stare could freeze the hearts of hardened criminals. How should I address him? By his title, or just his name? Did he have a title? What was his name?

In the end it was he who broke the silence.

'Gentlemen, thank you for coming so quickly. Please, come in.' He pushed himself up in the bed and smoothed down his hair. 'I'm sorry to get you out at this time of night. It was the doctor really – when I telephoned him he was quite adamant that an ambulance should be dispatched.'

'You don't have to apologize,' I said. 'The time doesn't make any difference to us. Why exactly did you call the doctor?'

He pulled on a pair of spectacles. 'Well, I have been

345

troubled all evening by a persistent pain in my chest. The funny thing is that since calling for you it seems to have subsided.'

'You mean it's gone completely?'

'Yes, I suppose it has. You must think I'm a bit of a fraud.'

It was novel to hear a judge describe himself as a fraud, but I wasn't going to argue the point. Instead, I encouraged him to describe his symptoms in more detail.

If I'd worried he might be something of an ogre, I needn't have. There wasn't a hint of affectation about him, just the self-deprecating charm of a gentleman from a world I seldom enter. His name was Andrew, and he continued to express his regret at inconveniencing us in a clipped, friendly voice that put me in mind of a leading man from a nineteen-forties movie.

'Indigestion, that's probably all it was. You must have more deserving patients to deal with. Thank you very much for coming – we must sort you out a cup of tea before you leave.'

When we eventually persuaded him that a trip to hospital might be a wise precaution he agreed gracefully.

'Well, you're the experts, and I suppose one has to bow to your greater knowledge, but . . .'

The oxygen mask silenced any other thoughts he may have had on the subject. As I wrapped him in a blanket, Larry eased a pair of slippers over his gnarled feet.

After the judge's bedchamber, our next port of call brought us back into what Mike might call the real world, a place where graciousness and respect are pretty thin on the ground. In fact, the case held echoes of Tom and the social club, though this time I had a certain amount of sympathy for the patient. The building was in the city centre and had probably once been the head office of a bank or insurance company. It still dealt with money, albeit the kind that passes across gambling tables.

Was it unreasonable to assume that, after making a 999 call, someone would be waiting to meet us? I didn't think it was, but we were left feeling about as welcome as a couple of Jehovah's Witnesses when we walked into the foyer. The only other people there were two men in evening suits standing by the reception desk. They saw us come in but, after an initial glance, continued their conversation. After a few moments the smaller of the two gathered some papers from the desk and headed towards the swing doors leading into the club proper. Larry put his bag down heavily.

'Hello. Excuse me ... has someone called for an ambulance?'

The short man looked over and, without breaking stride, spoke to his companion. 'Johnny, look after these two, will you.'

He might have been referring to a couple of draymen looking for the cellar.

Johnny fitted his thumbs into his waistcoat pockets

and regarded us from a face that not even his mother could have loved. He was a big man and, despite being the wrong side of forty and running to fat, presented an intimidating figure.

'All right, lads? Come and sign in, and I'll take you through.'

'Sign in?' Larry was incredulous. 'What are you on about? We're not here for a game of bloody blackjack!'

'Don't make no difference, everyone signs in. It's the law.'

He followed up this statement with a look that said the conversation was over. Larry was having none of it though. Being a similar height to Johnny, he walked over and looked him in the eye.

'We're not signing in! Have you got that? Now, where's the patient?'

Johnny drew himself up even taller and said, 'I've asked you nicely, now just sign in.'

The ludicrous implication that he wasn't going to ask so nicely a second time incensed Larry.

'We're not signing anything. Now take us to the patient, or you and I are going to fall out.'

I don't know exactly what he meant by that, and I never did find out because at that moment the first man came back.

'Is there a problem here?'

'Yes, boss. This pair won't sign in.' Johnny kept his eyes fixed on Larry as he spoke. The manager took on a conciliatory tone.

'Come on, lads, just sign the book.'

'No,' Larry said, his eyes locked with Johnny's.

The manager regarded the pair of them and sighed. 'OK, follow me.'

I was tempted to stick out my tongue at Johnny as we passed, but something told me not to bother.

The atmosphere inside the club was muted, with just the occasional voice rising above the background murmur. Gaming tables, mostly roulette and blackjack, stretched to the far side of the room where an expanse of wall-to-wall velvet curtain met the floor. As the manager led us on a circuitous route that kept us well away from the tables, I took the opportunity to ask the obvious question.

'So what's going on? Who have we come for?'

'It's Kerry, one of our croupiers. She got herself involved in a bit of unpleasantness with a punter, so we took her off the table and told her to take five and chill.' He broke off to acknowledge a passing customer, using craven body language that would have made Uriah Heep wince. Then, switching off the smile, he said, 'Next thing I know, she's throwing a wobbly in the toilets.'

'A wobbly?' I repeated.

'You know, getting all worked up. Fainting and stuff.'

'Oh, right,' I said, dubiously.

Then, by way of clarification, he added, 'You know how some women can behave when you give them a bit of a bollocking.'

He didn't hesitate at the padded door to the ladies' toilets but led us straight in. Kerry was sitting in front of a small vanity table clutching a hanky while one of her colleagues stroked her hair reassuringly. She must have been in her mid-twenties and was wearing an ankle-length dress that alerted one to her figure without shouting about it. I knelt down beside her, introduced myself and asked what was wrong. She didn't look at me, but managed to gasp out a reply.

'Nothing.'

So that was the way it was going to be. I'd have to extract the details from her bit by bit. She was breathing about twice as fast as anyone else in the room, which left me in little doubt that this was the problem I should treat. Hyperventilating is remarkably common in young people, especially after some kind of emotional upset. If it gets out of hand it can leave the victim feeling very ill, and sometimes genuinely frightened for their life. So, quietly and patiently, I got her to talk through the way she felt, and what had led up to her 'collapse'. From her replies I drew two separate conclusions. One, she was confused and embarrassed by the whole thing, and two, the row with her boss had left her humiliated and upset. Neither reason was an excuse to call an ambulance, but if I wanted to blame anyone it would be the manager, who, to use her own whispered words, was a complete arsehole.

Her breathing returned to normal as we talked and, when I was quite confident she wouldn't want to go to hospital, I offered to take her. My confidence was misplaced.

She glanced at her boss, who was standing with his back to us by the open door redirecting ladies to the disabled toilets, and said, 'I still feel weak and dizzy, I think I should have a check-up.'

'OK, Kerry,' I said, 'let's get you on your feet then.'

She stood up, but her legs wobbled and she flopped back down on to the chair. I can't say this came as much of a surprise; after all, being wheeled out would lend more credence to her plight. Larry must have seen it coming and had unfolded our chair in readiness for Kerry to edge on to. This done, I put a blanket over her exposed shoulders and we were ready to go.

Larry wheeled her towards the door, where he was forced to stop behind the manager.

'Excuse me . . . coming through.'

The manager turned with a look of mild surprise. 'Oh, she's going to hospital then?'

'That's the idea,' Larry said.

He rubbed his chin thoughtfully but didn't make any attempt to move.

'Er . . . look, do you think you could give it five minutes, ten at most?'

'Give what five minutes?'

'The club's just about to shut. I would appreciate it if you could hang on till the punters have gone.'

'Tell me you're not serious.' Larry seemed genuinely mystified.

'What's a few minutes? It's not going to go down too well with the punters to see one of the girls being wheeled through the gaming area.'

'I told you he was an arsehole,' Kerry whispered.

Larry went red in the face. 'Sorry, we're leaving now. If you'd stand aside please.'

The manager scowled. 'You've had an attitude on you since you walked through the door. One of your bosses is a member here. Just keep it in mind . . . I know people.'

Thinking of my new friend, Andrew the judge, I said, 'Well, you're not the only one who knows people. Now please, we would like to come past.'

Thirty seconds later we were back out in the foyer pushing Kerry purposefully towards the door. Johnny was giving Larry a truly evil eye and as we made our way down the steps I could feel the manager's gaze boring into the back of my head. I couldn't think what we had done to deserve all the flak, but I did know one thing – Larry and I wouldn't be applying for membership in the near future.

Chapter Twenty-two

'You don't expect me to go up there, do you?' I said.

The fireman followed my gaze upwards.

'It's strong enough, the workmen use it all the time. If you give me your right hand, my mate will take the other. I'll go first, you in the middle and my mate behind. Keep your back to the wall and we'll all just edge up together. There won't be any problems.'

I was horrified at this new twist. The dangerous ascent was one thing, but being seen holding hands with two firemen simply wasn't going to happen. I looked at him carefully in case it was his idea of a joke, then said, 'You're serious, aren't you? Well, you can forget it . . . I'm not holding hands with you, or your mate!'

'Sorry, but you've got no choice. I've had my orders. It's the only way you'll be allowed to go up.'

It was the first time I'd had any dealings with the fire brigade and it didn't take me long to discover the futility of arguing with one of them. A fireman who's had his orders . . . has had his orders. Eventually I gave up trying and, oozing as much bad grace as I could muster, held out my hands. I sensed rather than saw Larry's grinning face as I looked up at what was left of the staircase.

We were standing in the rubble-strewn entrance hall of a three-storey Victorian house that was being gutted prior to renovation. A gang of workmen had ventured into the roof space to remove the slates, then turned their attention to a brick chimney stack. It seemed that an overenthusiastic blow from a sledgehammer had brought the whole stack down on top of one of them. The fire brigade had arrived first and found the patient to be stable and conscious, though somewhat bruised and battered. It was when he complained of back pain that they decided to call us.

At first, I was confused. I don't claim to know anything about demolition, but I'd have thought it logical to start at the top of the building and work down. This wasn't the way they'd seen it; they'd started at the bottom and then worked their way up. As a result, the lower floors had been stripped bare and most of the interior fittings were missing, including the stairs. All that was left of them was a ragged ledge of wood running up the wall and sticking out about eighteen inches.

Health and safety was more a concept than a reality back in the seventies, leaving me with little choice but to put my faith in the firemen as we edged upwards. It wasn't difficult to ignore the drop ... I was too embarrassed by my predicament to worry about such trifles. What must I have looked like hand in hand with two firemen towering above me in their big yellow helmets? I prayed there wasn't a photographer from the *Evening Mail* down below. I could imagine a photo on the front page, along with the caption: 'INTREPID FIREMEN GUIDE AMBULANCE WORKER IN RACE TO SAVE STRICKEN BUILDER'. My life at the Street wouldn't be worth living if something like that appeared in the paper. I would have to emigrate.

We made it unscathed to the roof space and carefully picked our way over the rotting boards and exposed joists to the injured man. He'd been knocked about but, other than pain in the centre of his lower back, he hadn't sustained any worrying injuries. Hopefully it was just bruising, but we couldn't take any chances and had to treat for the worst. This meant keeping him flat and getting him into the Neil Robinson stretcher where he would be immobilized and could be moved safely. The problem was that the stretcher was on the ambulance, and the ambulance was thirty feet below us. There didn't seem to be any easy way to get the stretcher up, and even if we managed it there was certainly no way down. I turned to one of the firemen, only to be interrupted immediately.

'Don't worry, it's sorted.'

As he spoke, a movement behind his shoulder caught my eye. Larry's head was slowly appearing over the parapet. Its upward progress halted for a moment, then, in a series of jerky movements, it rose higher and allowed the rest of his body to come into view.

It was a sight that lingered in my memory for quite some time, even though the explanation proved mundane. He was standing on the platform of what is by far the most spectacular piece of equipment used by the fire brigade: the Snorkel. It's a long, hinged hydraulic arm anchored to a hefty six-wheeled vehicle. The arm can be ingeniously manoeuvred in seemingly any direction or at any angle desired by the operator. At the far end of this arm is a platform from where water is launched into a burning building. Its other function is that of rescue; it can reach up tall buildings, allowing people to be plucked to safety from windows and roofs. I'd always hoped that one day I'd get to take a ride on one, but so far the opportunity had eluded me. I wouldn't get a better chance than this, and was determined to stick close to my patient.

The platform swung across towards us and came to rest with a hiss. Larry nonchalantly stepped off, holding the stretcher, as if this means of arrival was an everyday event. He winked at me and asked if I'd managed to get the fireman's phone number. I'd expected some kind of jibe and, ignoring him, gave a brief explanation of what was needed. It took only minutes to get the injured workman carefully trussed up and ready to be loaded on to the Snorkel. I stepped on to the trembling platform, followed by a couple of firemen carrying the patient. There was a golden rule I'd heard more than once on station: never carry anything if there's a fireman around to carry it for you. There was no room for Larry, which was a shame, but I knew a fireman would hold his hand tightly on the way back down.

A shudder went through the metal floor beneath me and we were off, swinging out and away from the building. As I stood holding the railings, the breeze playing in my hair, I felt like the captain on the bridge of his ship. Now was the time for cameras: this would be a rather fine front-page picture for the evening paper.

Another ride on the Snorkel followed hot-foot after the first. We were told little more than that a gardener had been injured in the grounds of a large, detached house in Handsworth. A clue that there might be a little more to the case presented itself when we rounded the corner and spotted the Snorkel parked under a tree with its hydraulic arm half-buried in the canopy above. Howard and I looked at it curiously and, after a mental shrug of the shoulders, pulled into the drive with the intention of searching for the gardener. It was when we started walking towards the back garden that the fire officer called after us as if addressing a couple of schoolboys.

'Hey! Where are you two going?'

I didn't care much for his tone, but it was H, ever the diplomat, who answered.

'A gardener's been injured. We're going round the back to look for him.'

The fireman rolled his eyes. 'And what, pray, do you think we're doing here?'

This time the fireman's attitude got to H and although it was now obvious the presence of the fire brigade wasn't coincidental, he chose to be obtuse.

'I haven't a clue. Are you picking conkers?'

The officer glared at him, and pointed upwards. 'Your patient is in the tree.'

We looked up into the greenery. There he was, straddling a stout branch with a fireman in bright yellow leggings perched beside him. They were chatting as if waiting for a bus.

'So that's our gardener, is it? What's wrong with him, and what's he doing up a tree?' H asked.

'He's a tree surgeon. When he cut through one of the branches it slipped back on him and broke his arm. We can't get the platform in close enough, so we're going to have to lower him down, but his arm needs splinting first . . . That's where you come in.'

'So it was you lot who called for us?' H considered this for a moment. 'Don't get me wrong, I'm not trying to be funny or anything, but didn't you think it worth mentioning that the casualty was twenty feet up a horse-chestnut tree?'

The fireman chewed his lip. 'Which one of you is going up?'

'He is.' Howard was pointing at me.

Once on the Snorkel platform I was told to put on a safety harness. This rankled. I'd spent half my childhood in trees and the idea of being encumbered by a harness was, in my eyes, ridiculous, especially as the fireman already in the tree wasn't wearing one. Orders are orders though, and once raised as far as the branches would allow, I climbed over the railing and into the foliage, trailing a rope behind me. When I reached the patient a look of acute embarrassment ebbed through his otherwise tough exterior.

'Sorry about this, mate. I'm a total prat.'

I warmed to him immediately. 'Don't be silly . . . accidents happen.'

'Yeah . . . but not to me. This is going to keep me off work for weeks.' He held up his arm and winced.

I winced with him. The U-bend between his wrist and elbow was the worst I'd seen since being subjected to some pretty gruesome photos at training school.

'Well, it's broken all right,' I said in as nonchalant a tone as I could manage, and eased myself into a more comfortable position on the branch beside him. 'It'll feel a hell of a lot better when the splint's on.'

And I wasn't far wrong in that prediction. He visibly relaxed when the bones were held firmly in place and was ready to be bound in the harness that would lower him earthwards. There was a problem, however. There was only one harness, and I was wearing it. It was a silly situation that surely must have been foreseen, but I didn't detect any embarrassment on the part of the officer when he shouted through the branches that I should take it off and pass it over. Down below, H had set up the stretcher in such a position that the patient could be lowered straight on to it. I clung to the nearest branch like a spider-monkey and watched as the firemen played out the rope. The patient rotated slowly on the way down but landed neatly on the stretcher accompanied by a drizzle of early autumn leaves. Howard raised a thumb in my direction and I clambered back through the tree to the Snorkel platform.

Back on the ground the fire officer was beaming.

'Well! That went like clockwork, lads. It just goes to show that the two services can work well together when we make the effort. In fact, I'm in a mind to send a letter of commendation to your bosses.' He took out a notepad. 'What are your names?'

We gave him the information and a minute later he and his crew were gone in a cloud of diesel. I was elated. As I saw it, this would be the first entry in a portfolio that one day would be crammed with endorsements proclaiming me to be the long-awaited messiah the ambulance service craved. I could see medals being pinned to my chest by chief ambulance officers barely able to contain their emotions. My moment had arrived. But, unfortunately, the letter of praise didn't. I waited for it like a child anticipating Christmas Day, only for my hopes to be dashed and replaced by a deep feeling of umbrage.

I'd always been slightly mystified when my colleagues sneeringly referred to firemen as Trumptons, zombies or squirters. When I gave it some thought, I realized I'd never heard a word of praise or admiration for the work they carried out. I wouldn't say there was actual animosity between the two services; it was more a mutual disdain that had started a few years before I joined. What had been the Birmingham Fire and Ambulance Service was split into two separate entities, each going its own merry way. Quite why an antagonism developed is unclear to me, but the anecdotes I heard concerning firemen were at best negative, and more often than not designed to make them look foolish. Mike was fond of recalling the time he'd been called out to an accident involving a black cab. The driver's door had been crushed and two firemen were cutting away at it when the ambulance arrived. Mike wandered round to the near side of the vehicle and, seeing it was undamaged, extricated the 'trapped' cabbie with minimal fuss. So intent were the firemen in their work that they didn't notice, and were still hammering away at the door when the patient was loaded into the ambulance.

I felt vaguely uncomfortable about the bad blood between the services. We had a great working relationship with the police, but every time I made a friendly overture to a fireman I was invariably rebuffed, while picking up some sideways looks from my colleagues. In a way, I was quite pleased when the fire officer reneged on his promise; it gave me a personal axe to grind in any firemen-bashing conversation. The thing that irked us more than anything else though was their fondness for self-advertisement – or public relations, as it would now be called. They were masters at it while we were quite content to wait for our reward in heaven. A pretty good example of their ability to make something out of nothing, even if it meant stretching the truth about as far as it could be stretched, occurred not long after I'd clambered about in the horse-chestnut tree.

Steve and I had been called to stand by at a house fire late one evening. There hadn't been anyone home when the blaze started, and our job was to hang around in case one of the firemen hurt himself. We'd been there about ten minutes when a fireman emerged from the eddying smoke dragging a large black dog by its hind legs. He picked his way across the maze of water hoses criss-crossing the street while the dog's head bumped and flopped over each obstacle. Probably thinking it to be dead, he then abandoned it unceremoniously on the grass verge before disappearing back into the smoke. Steve and I walked over to have a look. The poor old thing was a sorry sight with his impossibly huge tongue lolling out on to the grass. He wasn't dead though. His chest rose a short way only to collapse prematurely, sending wisps of smoke curling from his mouth. The eyes stared rigidly ahead as if all his remaining energy was bent on fighting for his life.

We had to try and help, so we taped two oxygen masks together, placed them over his muzzle, turned up the flow to maximum, and waited to see what would happen. Five minutes later the dog's eyes became more focused and the lolling tongue somehow managed a slow retreat back into his mouth. We were quietly pleased, and as we sat there with the oxygen running a woman came over carrying a kitten. She handed it to me and I automatically took it into my arms as she bent down over the dog.

'Poor old Andrew,' she said, tickling his ear. 'How are you doing, darling? Who's had a nasty fright then?' The dog's tail lifted and dropped twice in response. She looked at me. 'Oh, isn't he a love? Is he going to be all right?'

'Yes, I hope so,' I said, trying to disentangle the kitten from a loose thread on my sleeve.

'That's good.' She turned back to the dog. 'We wouldn't want to lose you, would we, Andrew?' This elicited another tail thump. Satisfied, the woman walked off.

'Hey! What about this?' I held up the cat, but she was gone.

'I don't believe it!' Steve said. 'She thinks we're the bloody RSCPA.'

I assumed the kitten was another refugee from the house but on reflection he seemed too lively, and when I sniffed his fur there was no smell of smoke. Wherever he'd come from, it wasn't the fire. I now found myself with a kitten determined to shred my jacket, and a dog that was resolutely trying to get to its feet. What were we going to do with them? We couldn't take them with us, and when I offered custody to a passing fireman he just smiled and pointed out that we were the medics. We were saved when an elderly lady wandered over and volunteered to look after the animals. She lived in the neighbouring house and would keep them safe until their owners returned. The last we saw of our charges was the kitten in the woman's arms and Andrew staggering along beside her like an old man on his way home from the pub.

The next afternoon I had to smile, and give game, set and match to the fire brigade. All was quiet in the mess-room when Steve suddenly sat up in his chair and squawked, 'Bastards!' He was staring intently at the evening newspaper. 'I can't believe what I'm looking at . . . Of all the nerve!'

'Let's see then.' I got up from my chair. Steve held up the paper. Dominating the front page was a large photo of a fireman. He had a silly grin on his face and in the crook of his arm he held his upturned yellow helmet. Peeping over the brow was the cute little kitten from the previous night. The caption read something like 'SAVED FROM INFERNO – EIGHT LIVES LEFT!'

The accompanying article went on to describe how the cat had been rescued and then resuscitated by the firemen. Complete nonsense. It's true that Andrew couldn't be described as a beast overburdened with photogenic qualities, but that was no reason to deny him his moment of fame by substituting the kitten. There was no mention of our heroic role either; we'd been airbrushed from history.

'Bastards!' Steve repeated. 'Look, the picture's been taken in daylight. They must have gone back this morning with a photographer and sent the picture to the paper themselves! Can you believe it?'

Frankly, I could.

I had to get used to the fact that when the ambulance service was involved in an incident that made it into the press, the casualties would be described as 'arriving' at hospital with little or no mention of what had been done for them or, for that matter, who'd taken them there. This state of affairs was more or less accepted by everyone but, in those early days, I felt aggrieved from time to time – so much so that I plucked up the courage to tackle the station manager in the corridor one day and ask why we didn't get more credit. He was genuinely bemused by the question.

'Credit? You're doing the job you're paid to do, aren't you?'

'Well, yes, but . . .'

'You don't give a postman credit for delivering letters, do you?'

'Well, no, but . . .'

'So what's so special about you?'

'Well, nothing, I suppose.'

'There you go then. It's when you don't do your job

you'll hear from me. Now, for goodness' sake, son, get a grip.'

He wasn't alone in this attitude; it ran throughout the service and in time I came to see it as a rather healthy one. It could be a tough job, but I'd chosen it and it was up to me to get on with it.

Chapter Twenty-three

About a mile from Henrietta Street there's a row of small bungalows purpose-built for the elderly to live out their remaining years in safety and comfort. During the day an on-site warden keeps a discreet eye on them, and at night they have an emergency intercom system. It's a good arrangement for the old folk, allowing them control over their everyday lives in the knowledge that their security and well-being are catered for. Those up to it can even do a little gardening if they care to. The place is festooned with hanging baskets in the summer and the flowerbeds are always diligently tended. It was a particularly warm and pleasant September evening when Howard and I blundered into this neat little world, setting off a sad, irreversible chain of events.

Two ladies were working side by side pruning the roses when the elder caught the back of her hand on a thorn. For a younger person the injury would have been nothing more than an annoyance but for the old lady it was rather nasty. Her parchment-like skin split and parted, leaving the back of her hand red raw. She was led back into the bungalow, from where, much against her wishes, a neighbour called for an ambulance. We arrived to find her dwarfed in a large armchair, nursing a cup of tea. She looked up at us, her face aglow with a confident smile.

'Two nice young men. Aren't I the lucky one!' She put down the cup. 'They really shouldn't have called you. I told them not to, but they would insist.'

'Don't worry, it's no trouble,' I said. 'Anyway, we're here now so you might as well tell me what you've been up to.'

'I've been careless, look.' She held out her bloodied hand to be inspected.

'How on earth did you manage to do that?' I asked.

'I caught it on a Centifolia Bullata.' She knew the reaction this would get.

'You caught it on a what?'

'A Centifolia Bullata . . . it's a rose. It was silly of me, but there's no fool like an old fool.'

'Ivy's ninety, you know.' Her friend had taken up a matronly stance behind the chair. 'She's got all her marbles and she's as fit as a butcher's dog.'

I didn't doubt it for a moment.

I crouched down to her level and took a closer look at the injury, then wound a bandage round her hand.

'There you go, done and dusted.'

'Oh, thank you.' She laid a bony hand on the back of mine. 'It feels better already.'

Her charm, and the undeniable twinkle in her eye, made me smile.

'OK then, let's get your door keys and we'll pop you down to the hospital.'

She looked at me in amusement. 'What! For a little thing like this? Don't be so silly. What we all need now is a cup of tea.'

She was on her feet making for the kitchen before I could stop her. Her friend, who must have been well into her eighties, headed her off at the door and, ignoring the protests, led her back to the chair.

'It's quite a nasty wound,' I said. 'It might get infected. It needs to be properly cleaned and dressed. You might even need a tetanus jab.'

My words didn't cut any ice.

'I've never been to a hospital in my life, and wild horses couldn't drag me there now!'

The thought of her tiny six-stone frame battling against wild horses made me smile again.

'They won't keep you long. It'll only be an hour or so and then, Bob's your uncle . . . you'll be back home.'

'Yes,' she said, 'and Fanny might well be your aunt, but I'm still not going.'

Howard, who'd been standing quietly in a corner, stepped forward.

'Ivy, there's nothing to worry about. The hospital's

only round the corner, you'll be back home before you know it.'

Though well intended, his intervention didn't help. Ivy's voice went up a couple of octaves.

'No. I don't want to sound rude, but I'm not going and that's the end of it!'

A trace of fear was mixed with the defiance. Seeing she was becoming upset, H backed off. We were changing from 'nice young men' into a couple of bullies. I was reminded of a poster on the training school wall featuring the cartoon figure of a snarling wolf wearing an ambulance uniform. Underneath was written: 'Remember . . . this is what you may look like to a child.' The message was simple but effective. We weren't exactly dealing with a child, but her reaction made me feel like the wolf. I put a hand on her shoulder.

'Listen, Ivy. We're not taking you to hospital if you don't want to go, it was just an offer. You're the boss.'

It seemed to work; the smile returned and she placed her hand back on my arm.

'I know you're only thinking of me, and I'm not ungrateful, but I've never been to hospital and I can't bear the idea of going now.'

I wasn't going to push it any further.

'Don't worry. I tell you what, shall we get your doctor to come out and give you a tetanus jab?'

At this point, fate played its card in the form of two policemen. They'd been passing the bungalow and, spotting the ambulance parked outside, decided to look in and see what was going on. They strolled into the lounge unannounced. One was tall and thin, the other tall and fat. Ivy looked across at them and her face crumpled.

'Oh dear me! Policemen . . . I'm not going!'

Her grip tightened on my arm as H quietly explained the situation to the officers. The thinner of the two, probably thinking he'd show us a thing or two about the gentle art of persuasion, strode forward. Towering over Ivy, he spoke loudly.

'Now, now. What's all this? Why don't you want to go to hospital with the ambulance men . . .'

It was too much for her. She buried her head in my shoulder and in a quavering voice begged to be left alone. I rolled my eyes to the ceiling in exasperation and the policeman, embarrassed, retreated, leaving me to repair the damage. After a few moments trying to placate her, I became aware that she was leaning rather heavily on me, so I moved position to speak to her directly. Without the support of my shoulder, her head lolled back against the cushion, her eyes staring fixedly somewhere above me.

I checked her pulse. There wasn't one, and the world around seemed to go into slow motion as I struggled with the enormity of what had happened.

'Get her on the floor!' Howard's voice brought me back. Cradling her head gently, and with Howard's help, I lowered her to the carpet and checked again. H snatched the bag and mask from its case, connected it to the oxygen and began rhythmically inflating her lungs while I started cardiac compressions. Her ribcage creaked as I pressed down, leaving me appalled at her frailty. Too much pressure and her ribs would snap like sun-dried twigs; not enough pressure and there would be no benefit in what I was doing. As we worked, Howard looked round at the policemen now standing on the far side of the room.

'Go and get our stretcher!' He didn't exactly shout at them, but they flew from the room as if fired from a gun. They were back with the stretcher in less than a minute, gouging a chunk of wood from the doorframe in their agitation. Together we lifted Ivy on to the cot and dashed from the bungalow, past the roses, to the ambulance. The hospital was only two or three minutes away.

We transferred her swiftly on to the Casualty trolley and stepped back as the hospital staff took over. A doctor asked me how old she was. I told him.

'Ninety, not a bad innings.' He sniffed.

The inference was clear. I started to tell him what a good quality of life she enjoyed, but he'd lost interest and moved away. There was an air of inevitability about the outcome; no one expected or even hoped for anything other than the doctor in charge calling it a day. After a few minutes' effort, he did so.

'Thanks very much, everybody. That's it, I'm afraid.'

Protocols had been satisfied. A sheet was pulled over Ivy and the staff started to drift from the room. I stared at the shape on the bed. It was all unreal; a quarter of an hour ago she'd been offering me a cup of tea. She should be in her garden pruning the roses or, at worst, sitting in her living room nursing a sore hand. We'd gone to her aid with the best of intentions; a simpler, more routine case would be difficult to imagine. Where had it all gone wrong? It wasn't our fault . . . was it?

If it was merited, H liked nothing better than to talk through a case afterwards. His gregarious enthusiasm for the job always left him asking questions of himself, not to mention answering mine. This time it was different. He was morose, and didn't seem to have any appetite to reveal his thoughts other than to say, 'If we'd left her alone she'd still be alive.' He didn't criticize the police officers, or try to justify our own actions. Instead, he seemed to be looking inwards at what I'm sure he perceived to be personal failure. His dark mood was in such contrast to the Howard I knew that it left me wondering if these 'old hands' really did shrug off tribulations quite as easily as I'd imagined.

The manner of Ivy's death didn't just put a break on my burgeoning confidence; it marked the start of a dark period that would test my fortitude. Things had been ticking along so nicely over the previous weeks. Fuelled by small successes, my confidence had been on the way up, which was just as well as my twelve-month probationary period had drawn to an end. The boss marked the occasion with a four-second speech before thrusting the coveted Millers Certificate in my direction. The Millers was, in its day, the ambulance service's official recognition of competence. I was of course delighted to reach this milestone but, as ever, there was a sting in the tail. Being fully qualified meant I'd be expected to shoulder more responsibility and, heaven forbid, occasionally oversee new recruits. Not an unreasonable expectation from management's point of view, but I knew it would take more than a year to shake off my reliance on the older, wiser heads around me.

It was rare for two relatively inexperienced people to be crewed together. When it did happen it was usually the result of the rota being understaffed due to holidays or sickness. As things worked out, I didn't have to wait long to be thrown in the deep end. Howard had called in sick for the night shift, which left the boss phoning around trying to badger someone into coming in on overtime. I was blissfully unaware of the developments when I strolled into the messroom, a situation Larry was only too keen to rectify.

'I see you're going to be in charge tonight.'

'In charge? I don't remember applying for promotion.' I dropped into a chair, only vaguely interested in what he was leading up to.

Larry pretended to search for the right words. 'It's not exactly what you'd call promotion. It's more a case of you being given the opportunity to pass on some of your extensive knowledge.'

I paused in the act of reaching for a nearby news-paper and regarded him with suspicion.

'What?'

'Howard's gone sick,' Larry continued. 'They've crewed you up for the night with Brian from A shift. He's out in the garage checking the motor.'

'Brian? Never heard of a Brian,' I said, trying to keep any trace of alarm from my voice.

'You must have seen him around,' Larry said. 'He started a few weeks ago. Little fella covered in acne? Looks like a dormouse with a guilty secret.'

The air seemed to have been sucked from my chest. I had indeed seen him around. He was the latest arrival at the Street and you didn't need to be Sherlock Holmes to recognize it. He wore the haunted look of someone who'd woken in the Twilight Zone and come to the horrified realization that there was no hope of escape. He was at the mercy of the Henrietta Street ruffians, any one of whom could make him jump out of his skin by just saying boo. Word had drifted back from his shift that they were in despair of ever knocking him into shape. I had to stay calm. Larry mustn't know I was on the point of bolting for the window and jumping out. I stood up and stretched lazily.

'I'd better go and see what he's up to. He should be making the tea, not messing about on the ambulance.'

I made my way out to the garage bent under the weight of true responsibility for the first time in my life. It wasn't fair. It was too soon. How could I be expected to act as nursemaid when I was barely weaned myself? Thoughts of all the things that could and probably would go wrong poured through my head in an unstoppable torrent. My pulse quickened. This was the night when I'd end up attending a crash on the M6 ... it had to be. I stopped walking. I must be positive. It was a Tuesday; in all likelihood it would be a quiet night with only a few routine cases. I tried to take comfort in thinking back over some of the more difficult jobs I'd been out to, but it didn't work. There'd always been someone's coat tails for me to hide behind.

Brian was bent over an oxygen cylinder trying to break the seal when I spoke to him from the back doors. He swung round, dropping the key with a clatter.

'Oh, sorry.' He leaned down to retrieve it. 'I didn't realize you were there.'

His large, brown eyes were wide, and I felt a pang of sympathy.

'I didn't mean to creep up on you. I'm Les. It seems we're crewed up tonight.'

'Yes, I hope you don't mind.'

'Mind? Why should I mind?'

'It's just that I'm a bit new and haven't quite got the hang of things yet.'

The news wasn't exactly a revelation, but at least he was honest.

'Don't worry about that.' Then I added, a little

piously, 'We all had to start once. If you've got any questions, just fire away.'

'Thanks for that, I'm sure I'll have plenty. What do you want me to do tonight, by the way – drive or attend?'

It was a question I'd never faced before, and I gave the answer I'd been receiving for the past year.

'You better attend . . . you'll never learn this job sitting in the front.' With that I left him to his checks and returned to the messroom, slightly weak at the knees.

Our first call-out was to a notorious pub in Nechells, arguably the roughest district in the city. In former days it had been a poor but basically decent, working-class community, which was allowed to drift downwards on the back of neglect and deprivation. During the sixties space was found among the terraced streets to throw up three-storey blocks of flats, the blueprints of which could only have come from one of Stalin's five-year plans. Looking more like military barracks than homes, they were gradually filled with an army of disaffected and unemployable families who turned the streets into no-go areas after dark to such effect that even cats went about in twos. The job description we'd been given was 'man assaulted'. This hardly came as a surprise, and as we made our way through the city I warned Brian to stay close and be careful, especially if the police weren't there.

Our patient was spreadeagled on the ground near the

pub's only entrance. I knew he was dead before I opened my door. There was an ominous stillness about the body, a stillness that conveyed its message even to those who might never have seen it before. He was on his back, his shoulders on the pavement and his legs, one buckled under the other, resting on the steps of the building. People from the pub had gathered round, but none was closer than three feet. An invisible barrier separated the living from the dead. My stomach churned as I eased through the silent knot of bystanders and bent over the man. My first murder and, to all intents and purposes, I was on my own.

He was powerfully built, casually dressed and probably in his late twenties. There was a small but vivid bloodstain high up on his white T-shirt. His face was transfixed in death; mouth slack, eyes open, pupils fixed and dilated. There was no pulse. Lifting his T-shirt revealed two puncture wounds high up on the left side of his chest. In themselves they were small, innocuous even, but I'd seen their like before, albeit in people still alive. He'd been stabbed.

'He's not breathing, is he? What do you want me to do?' Brian was crouching beside me. I held his eye for the briefest moment.

'There's no pulse either. Start chest compressions while I get some air into him.'

I hit a problem straight away. The mixture of pure oxygen and air I was trying to force into his lungs via the bag and mask was escaping round the contours of his jaw. There was nothing impeding his airway but no matter how I tried, I couldn't get an effective seal. I felt hot and anxious; Mike wouldn't have had any trouble, what was I doing wrong? If I was failing in the basic task of inflating his lungs, what hope was there? Then Brian spoke again.

'I can't seem to do this.' He was looking at me, near panic etched in his face.

'What can't you do?' I snapped back, still wrestling with the bag and mask.

'The compressions, I can't seem to get enough power.'

'For Christ's sake!' I said in exasperation. 'Change over. See if you can get a seal with the mask and I'll have a go at his chest.'

I got in position and began what was intended to be a sequence of ten rapid downward thrusts just above his sternum.

With my first push I knew it was all over. His chest was as unyielding as a sandbag. I tried again with considerably more force but still couldn't make any impression. I hadn't seen or heard of anything like it before, and my mind raced as I tried to find a reason. From the position of the wounds there was every chance at least one blow had penetrated his heart. Could it be that its last few beats had made his chest cavity fill with blood? Had a major blood vessel been cut, with the same effect? A build-up of blood was the only possible explanation why his chest was rigid and his lungs wouldn't inflate. The lack of any significant external bleeding suggested his heart had stopped very soon after he'd been injured. I looked round and caught the eye of a bystander.

'How long is it since he collapsed?'

'I dunno. Fifteen, maybe twenty minutes.'

He must have been dead before we left the Street.

Car doors slammed nearby and I looked up as two police officers came over at a fast walk. One looked down at the body, then at me.

'Is it bad?'

'It's as bad as it gets. He's dead . . . stabbed, by the look of it.'

Even under the streetlights I could see his colour drain.

'Christ!'

Brian was still engrossed in his battle with the bag and mask as I leaned back from the body and stood up.

'You can forget that, Brian. There's nothing we can do for him.'

He looked up at me in surprise. 'I think I'm starting to get somewhere . . .'

As he squeezed the bag I could hear the hiss of air escaping over the man's face.

'No, you're not. Go and fetch a blanket from the ambulance and cover him up.'

'We're not taking him to hospital then?'

I suddenly felt tired. Taking responsibility for a decision like this wasn't something that came easy.

'No. It's a crime scene now. The police will want everything left as it is.'

More police cars arrived, their blue lights rhythmically bathing the lonely body on the ground. The growing crowd were persuaded to move back and as an officer began cordoning off the area Brian returned with a blanket, which he gently draped over the young man. With that done, we walked back to the ambulance together. I had to wait before getting through to Control on the radio. Not half a mile away another crew was calling for police assistance after running into trouble with a gang of youths throwing bottles at their ambulance. As we waited, Brian raised his hands.

'Look, I'm shaking.'

I glanced at him, slightly surprised at his willingness to reveal what most people would do their best to hide.

'Don't worry about it. It happens sometimes after an adrenalin rush.'

He regarded his hands a little longer, then dropped them back on his lap.

'I suppose you've seen this kind of thing a few times. Have you been to many murders?'

'No,' I said. 'This is my first.'

If he'd been a little more observant, he might have noticed I was sitting on my hands.

An intriguing postscript to this story unfolded a year later in the unlikely setting of my local pub. I was with my dog, Pip, a delightfully gregarious Staffordshire bull terrier who greeted anyone who happened through the door as a long-lost and dear friend. There weren't many who could resist her, not least a stranger who came into the bar one evening. He made a huge fuss of the dog and when they both eventually calmed down we started to chat. The conversation roamed over the subject of dogs and when that was exhausted I idly commented that I hadn't seen him in the pub before. He took a pull at his pint.

'I used to be a regular here, but I use the King's Arms these days. That's where I was tonight until some prat at the bar took out a knife and showed it off to his mates. There wasn't any trouble or anything, but I couldn't get out the place fast enough. I've had this kind of phobia about knives since my brother was killed by one.'

As a conversation stopper, it was a pretty good line. But that didn't matter; he seemed happy to continue without any prompts from me. As he described the circumstances of his brother's death my general unease began to turn to disquiet. Surely it couldn't be the same stabbing Brian and I had attended? It had taken place the previous year, which fitted. It happened in a Nechells pub, which also fitted. Then, as more of the story unfolded, the similarities became too overwhelming to be mere coincidence.

'This pub,' I said, tentatively. 'It wasn't the Dragon, was it?'

He looked at me sharply. 'How do you know that?'

I shifted in my seat, unsure what to say. There was no way of knowing how he'd react when he found out he was sitting next to the very person whose mission it had been to try and save his brother's life. But, then again . . . how could I not tell him?

I took a deep breath. 'I know because I was one of the ambulance crew who went out to your brother that night.'

His eyes widened and he stared at me long and hard.

'Are you serious? You wouldn't joke about something like this, would you?'

'Of course I wouldn't. It was a terrible night.' As I waited for his reaction I added, 'I'm sorry we couldn't help him.'

There were a few moments' silence and then he thrust his hand in my direction, which I took with relieved gratitude. We then fell into a prolonged discussion about what happened that night. I was able to bring a little clarity to his understanding of the scene, while he confirmed that the killer blow had indeed penetrated the heart and caused almost instantaneous death. He also said that the perpetrator had been caught and convicted, which pleased me greatly.

Our meeting happened many years ago but we remain friends to this day. In fact, just recently he sent a pint over to my table. When I asked why, I was told that it was to mark the anniversary of his brother's death.

Chapter Twenty-four

In many ways Jack Turner, the latest member of the shift, bucked the norm by settling in so well you'd have thought he'd been there for years. It's difficult to put my finger on exactly how he managed it, but maybe his confidence and mature understanding of the ways of the world had something to do with it. He was also wise. It wasn't by chance that he always deferred to the knowledge and experience of the others. Never once did he try to bluff his way through a work-related conversation, which always meant social death to anyone who did. But that was as far as his deference went. In every other respect he was his own man, not an easy trick to pull off in the strictly hierarchical world of Henrietta Street.

Something I couldn't understand was Jack's obvious fondness for Larry. Jack had a sophisticated and at times wicked sense of humour, which made it all the more odd to see him joining in the horseplay and practical jokes Larry thrived on. It was doubly baffling when you considered that Jack was usually to be found cosied up with a book, or working his way through the *Telegraph* crossword, something that rarely took him longer than twenty minutes. One evening Larry, being Larry, pushed Jack too far.

Jack was in a contemplative mood, content to sit in his chair with a book while the rest of us played cards. Larry, never happy seeing someone reading a book at the best of times, did his best to cajole him into joining us. When all failed, he saw it as a matter of principle to get Jack out of his chair, and began rolling sheets of newspaper into tubes and lightly knotting them. As each one was ready he threw it under Jack's seat as if preparing the kindling for a coal fire. All the while Jack feigned lack of interest and continued reading. Eventually he licked a finger before turning a page and said, in a lazy kind of way, 'If you light that paper, Larry . . . I'm going to hang you.'

Something in his tone made people look up.

That Larry chose to ignore the warning was, even by his foolishness standard, remarkable. We all knew Jack was capable of extraordinary and, where the recipient was concerned, damaging acts of violence. He still worked as a club bouncer on his nights off and, it must be pointed out, nightclub bouncers in the seventies were a very different kettle of fish from those of today. No yellow coats, identity cards and diplomas in anger management or negotiating skills for them. The only qualification they needed was the ability to drop an eighteen-stone man with a single blow. So when Larry threw a lit match on to the pile we all gave a little gasp of disbelief.

Not much happened at first. Jack didn't move as the dull orange flame rose almost apologetically from the curling newspaper and spread lazily to the sheets close by. An instant later the whole lot went up with a woomph. Jack was briefly silhouetted in its midst before leaping from the conflagration with such lightning speed that Larry barely had time to react. A hairy paw missed his throat by an inch and, acting purely on animal instinct, he shot into the corridor with Jack in close and determined pursuit. Steve grabbed the fire extinguisher from its hinge by the door and frantically blasted the flames, sending the burning embers into every corner of the room. Mike leaped from his chair to protect his precious snooker table while the rest of us stamped about on the dying flames, desperately trying to minimize the damage.

While we cursed and danced, the villain of the piece was evading capture out in the garage. There weren't many people who could outrun Larry, and Jack certainly wasn't one of them. He gave up after a few minutes and came back into the messroom carrying a length of rope he'd taken from one of the emergency rescue bags. We were too busy damping down and wiping sooty stains from the furniture to pay much attention as he resumed his seat and started to methodically fashion a hangman's noose. When it was finished he held it up and let it swing gently in his grasp. One by one we drifted over to admire his handiwork. As someone who could barely tie his own shoelaces, I was particularly impressed.

'Are you really going to hang Larry with it?' Steve asked with a smile.

Jack stood up and headed for the door. 'That's the general idea.'

Steve seemed unsure if he was joking or not, but played along.

'Can we give you a hand?'

'No. It's a one-man job.' And with that he headed off down the corridor to the garage.

A silence descended on the room until Mike broke it by asking who was working with Jack.

'I am,' I said.

'OK. The next job to come in is yours, regardless of where you are in the running order. Much as I'd like to see Larry strung up from the rafters, it might not be a good career move for Jack.'

'Not only that,' Steve said, 'just think of the reputation the Street would get.'

When the 999 came through some ten minutes later I scribbled down the details and went looking for Jack. He was wandering up and down the rows of parked ambulances, swinging the noose and calling Larry's name in a gentle, motherly kind of way. The garage, which is about half the size of a football pitch, offered

Larry plenty of hiding space. He was out there in the shadows somewhere, keeping very quiet indeed.

'Sorry to spoil the fun, Jack, but we've got a job.'

He turned and looked at me. 'We're not next out.'

'I'm afraid we are,' I said as I got into the cab. 'It's a woman collapsed in the street so we can't really hang around, if you'll excuse the pun.'

Jack brought the noose with him and threw it into the footwell.

'You're not thinking of hanging me with that, are you?' I asked as I swung the ambulance out on to the road.

'No, so long as you promise not to try and set me on fire.'

'What would you have done if you'd caught him?' I asked.

'I don't suppose we'll ever know now.' Then he smiled. 'I have to hand it to him. He's either very brave or very, very stupid.'

'I know which one I'd put my money on.'

'Well, stupid or not, he's not out of the woods yet.' Then, changing the subject, he asked, 'Where are we going?'

'Lozells.' I tried to sound blasé with the next bit. 'Apparently a naked woman's been spotted lying in the street.'

I turned into the cul-de-sac and straight away spotted her stretched out on the pavement. She was under a street lamp, stark naked as predicted, and smoking a cigarette. I dropped Jack off with a blanket and first aid bag and carried on down the street to turn the ambulance round. Jack was waiting for me when I returned.

'She doesn't seem to be hurt, but I'm telling you, she's one weird woman. Every time I try to put the blanket over her she just pulls it off.'

'What's she got to say for herself?' I asked.

'That's another thing. She won't say a word. I'm telling you, she's weird.'

'Oh well, let's see if I can get anywhere with her.'

I looked down at the contented face and wondered where to start.

'Hi, I'm Les. Can you tell me what's happened?'

Silence.

'Come on now. You have to talk to me and tell me what this is all about. Has someone hurt you?'

Silence.

'You must be cold. Where are your clothes?'

She took a long drag on her cigarette and blew a stream of smoke over my shoulder into the night sky. Not only did she refuse to speak; she wouldn't even acknowledge my existence. I'd been on the receiving end of similar treatment from girlfriends in the past, but this was a first as far as a patient was concerned.

The situation needed some thought. I wasn't able to check her sugar levels, but as her actions – casting aside the blanket and smoking the cigarette – were calculated in their execution, it seemed unlikely that diabetes was behind it. Drugs? I didn't think so. She had to be at least forty and, on the face of it, perfectly healthy. She wasn't showing any sign of distress or injury. On the contrary, she was the very picture of contentment and seemed happy to while away the time taking the occasional pull on her cigarette and regarding the stars above. My original fear that she'd been the victim of an assault began to fade.

I was scratching my head hoping for a flash of inspiration when Jack knelt down and said, as he draped the blanket over her again, 'You must be freezing out here in the cold. Why don't you come and sit in the ambulance where it's warmer?'

Slowly, she turned her eyes in his direction and fixed him with a cold stare. I wasn't sure if this was an encouraging sign or not, but I didn't have to wait long to find out. Rather than speak to him as I'd hoped, she took a long drag on her cigarette and deliberately blew a plume of smoke into his face. Then she grabbed the blanket and threw it across the pavement. As Jack patiently strolled off to retrieve it she took a fresh cigarette from the packet, lit it from the old one, and resumed her contemplation of the heavens.

It had been drummed into me that calling on the police to solve our problems was an admission of defeat. No matter how I looked at things though, there didn't seem much else I could do. The police have the power to take someone to a place of safety whether the patient likes it or not. We don't. Trying to physically force the woman on to her feet was out of the question; not least because she was naked, obviously unbalanced and, given the circumstances, had the potential to accuse us of anything. It was a shame. Everything would be so much easier, I thought, if we could sort it out here and now. Reluctantly, I turned to Jack as he draped the blanket over the woman for a third time.

'Well, I don't think we've any other option but to get the police here.'

My words lit a fuse under the woman. Without warning she leaped to her feet. The blanket fell to the ground and she marched, arms swinging and straight-backed like a guardsman, to the rear of the ambulance. Hardly believing our luck, I grabbed the blanket and followed her.

She was a big girl by anyone's standards, and the moonlight danced over her ample frame as she mounted the ambulance steps and threw herself heavily on to the stretcher. Once comfortable, she folded her arms, crossed her legs and took another long drag on her cigarette. So far I hadn't exercised any control whatsoever over events, but that didn't bother me: the immediate problem had been resolved. I threw Jack the keys and told him to get going before she had a change of heart. He closed the back doors and ran round to the front and a moment or two later we were off with a lurch. I placed the blanket over her yet again, but she straight away pulled it off and let it fall to the floor. I left it there and sat back in my seat to take stock.

The first thing I had to do was get the cigarette off her, and from the way things had gone so far I had the feeling it wasn't going to be particularly easy. There was a vomit bowl on the shelf and I picked it up to use as an ashtray.

'Can I have the cigarette please?' Getting no response, I tried a more light-hearted approach. 'We've got oxygen on board and you wouldn't want to blow us up, would you?' This earned me the same disconcerting stare she'd bestowed on Jack earlier. With her gaze remaining fixed on me, she lifted up the cigarette between forefinger and thumb, as if offering it to me. As I reached out, she reversed it between her fingers so the burning tip was pointing downwards and suddenly plunged it towards her stomach. I couldn't react in time to stop her. The lit end went into her navel and she pressed down, rotating it slightly, until it was out.

The whole thing was over in an instant, but it felt as if it had taken place in slow motion. Aghast at what she had done, I was on my feet gaping down at her, waiting for her reaction to the pain. It didn't come. She didn't appear to have felt a thing, but a spell seemed to have been broken. There was the hint of a smile on her face as she handed over the extinguished nub. I took it and, trying to ignore the smell of burned skin wafting up from the stretcher, stared down stupidly at her navel. I threw the nub out of the window and then, to cover my own confusion as much as anything else, I tore open a dressing and placed it on the burn, then replaced the blanket. With that done, I slumped back down into my seat and tried to come to terms with what had just happened. Eventually, I found something stupid to say.

'Why did you do that?' It was a question that would never be answered. But, as if woken from a trance, she became talkative. She told me her name and, ignoring my interruptions, started talking manically about her family without seeming to take a breath. She named her brothers, sisters, aunts, uncles, parents and grand-parents before giving me their ages and where they all lived. I gave up trying to stop her and listened patiently as she changed tack and began regaling me with anecdotes concerning her relatives, dead and alive. We hadn't got far to travel, but even so I learned a lot of things I didn't want to know about her extended family. She was carefully explaining the exact order in which some long-dead aunt always cooked the vegetables for Sunday lunch when we reached Casualty. An air of fatalism had descended on me by the time Jack opened the doors, and as we steered the stretcher past the late-night drunks infesting the waiting area I was still trying to sort the whole business out in my mind.

The triage nurse was sitting behind her desk and gave our patient a big smile. She, now the very picture of normality, beamed back at her. The nurse then turned to me and waited for information. The standard line when handing over a patient is to start with the chief complaint. Once that's established, we can move on to describe the circumstances and any general observations we may have. That's followed up with a rundown of the patient's medical history. I hesitated.

'Well?' said the nurse. 'I'm listening.'

Where to start? The woman's mental health problems were obviously legion, and the reason she was here. Physically, there was the burn, so I decided to get that out of the way first and then move on to the more complicated subject of her bizarre behaviour.

'Well, to start with, she's got a nasty cigarette burn on her navel . . .'

The nurse grimaced and cast a sympathetic look at the patient. 'Oh gosh, that sounds painful. How long ago did that happen?'

The woman considered the question. 'Oh, it can't be much more than ten minutes ago.' Then, looking at me for confirmation, she added, 'It was just after I got on the ambulance, wasn't it?'

The nurse threw me a quizzical look. 'Am I missing something here? She got burned *after* you picked her up?'

'No . . . well . . . yes, she did . . . but it wasn't quite that simple. I was trying to give her an ashtray but—'

The nurse interrupted. 'An ashtray? You've got ashtrays on the ambulances?'

'What? No! Of course not. I was trying to get her to use a vomit bowl as an ashtray—'

The nurse held up a hand. 'Hang on. Stop right there. Let's go back to the beginning, shall we . . . ?'

The bizarre case of the naked lady left me wondering whether to laugh or cry. I was still in a fragile state of mind after a run of depressing jobs, and to describe life on the ambulance service as a roller-coaster existence is something of an understatement. The highs and lows can follow each other with such bewildering speed that if you are to stay on your feet it's essential to roll with the punches. Miraculously, and despite plenty of wobbles along the way, I was still standing at the end of an eighteen-month battering. It was wonderful to know the path I'd taken almost on impulse had been the right one after all. It hadn't been an easy journey, and I'm the first to admit to the times when I've been left ruing the day I'd ever thought of joining the ambulance service, but such moments were fleeting.

And what of the future? Well, that was a question I don't remember being troubled by – my future was with the ambulance service. It was as simple as that. Ahead lay a blank canvas waiting to be coloured by characters and events I had no way of foreseeing or even imagining. I had barely sketched in the background, and leaving the rest unpainted was unthinkable. But I wasn't so naive as to dismiss all the tribulations and heartaches I would inevitably have to face; that would have been foolish. Tough times were lying in wait, no doubt about it, but such forebodings were tempered by the certain knowledge that the joys and triumphs would outweigh all else.

And had eighteen months spent caring for others revealed a compassionate side to my nature that had previously lain dormant? Well, I think that it had, and I proved it by performing my final humanitarian act of the night: when Jack was distracted, I spirited the noose from the ambulance and dropped it in a nearby bin. Thanks to me, Larry would live to fight another day.

Call the Ambulance!

Les Pringle

EXPLODING PRESSURE COOKERS, a thwarted wife's deadly revenge and transvestites in distress – manning an ambulance in the seventies kept you on your toes.

Having survived the rites of passage as a probationer, Les Pringle now has to face up to the reality of life as an ambulance man in seventies Britain. He does this with humour and fortitude – two qualities which are essential if he is to cope with cases ranging from the absurd to the heart rending.

From attending murder scenes to delivering babies . . . it's quite a life for Les, and one that he and his shift mates tread with warmth and humour in equal measure.

'He's a very engaging a writer . . . I cannot
recommend it enough'
Tom Reynolds, author of *Blood, Sweat and Tea*

9780552158534

Nobody in Particular

Cherry Simmonds

LOOKING BACK, BEING the youngest of nine children and a change of life baby, conceived and born on Merseyside during the war, was probably not the best start for my Mam or me . . .

Hand-on-heart honest, charming, occasionally tear-inducingly tragic but more often laugh-out-loud funny, *Nobody in Particular* is Cherry Simmonds' account of growing up on the back streets of Liverpool in the 50s and 60s, the youngest in a large, eccentric and sometimes exasperating Anglo-Irish family. Ruling the roost was Mam – menopausal and always saving for a divorce, or her own business, which ever was cheaper. And Dad – who when he wasn't in the pub could invariably be found in the outside lav practising the banjo, and her five brothers and four sisters – two died, three got married (which amounted to the same thing according to Mam) and National Service would take care of the rest . . .

Recalling the despondent, still-rationed post-war years as well as the heady, swinging 60s – when Liverpool suddenly found itself fashionable, put on the map by the Beatles, industrial strikes, and Liverpool FC winning the Cup – and full of memorable characters, this wonderfully delightful memoir brings a bygone yet still familiar and fondly remembered era to life.

9780553815283

Teacher, Teacher!

Jack Sheffield

MISS BARRINGTON-HUNTLEY took off her steel-framed spectacles and polished them deliberately. 'Mr Sheffield,' she said, 'after careful consideration we have decided to offer you the very challenging post of headmaster of Ragley School'.

It's 1977 and Jack Sheffield arrives at a small village primary school in North Yorkshire. Little does he imagine what the first year will hold in store as he has to grapple with:

Ruby, the 20 stone caretaker with an acute spelling problem

Vera, the school secretary who worships Margaret Thatcher

Ping, the little Vietnamese refugee who becomes the school's best reader and poet

Deke Ramsbottom, a singing cowboy, father of Wayne, Shane and Clint,

and many others, including a groundsman who grows giant carrots, a barmaid parent who requests sex lessons, and a five-year-old boy whose language is colourful in the extreme. And then there's beautiful, bright Beth Henderson, a deputy head, who is irresistibly attractive to the young headmaster . . .

'Heartbeat for teachers'
Fay Yeomans, *BBC RADIO*

9780552155281

Paperboy

Christopher Fowler

SUPERMAN, DRACULA, TREASURE *Island*, *The Avengers* ... when you're ten years old you can fall in love with any story, so long as it's a good one. But what do you do if you're growing up in a home without books? Christopher Fowler's childhood memoir captures life in suburban London through the eyes of a lonely boy who spends his days between the library and the cinema devouring novels, comics, cereal boxes – *anything* that might reveal a story. But it is 1960, and after fifteen years of post-war belt-tightening, his family's not quite ready to indulge a child cursed with too much imagination ...

Caught between an ever-sensible, exhausted mother and a DIY-obsessed father fighting his own demons, Christopher takes refuge in words. His parents try to understand their son's peculiar obsession but they fast lose patience with him – and each other. As the war of nerves escalates to include every member of the Fowler family, something has to give, but do the tough lessons of real life mean a boy must always let go of his dreams?

The memoir of a childhood at once eccentric and endearingly ordinary, this does for storytelling what Nigel Slater's *Toast* did for food.

'*Paperboy* is fabulous, and I hope it sells forever.'
Joanne Harris

9780553820096